T0197264

Rating Scales in Psychiatry

Peter Tyrer & Caroline Methuen

with a foreword by

Simon Gilbody

RCPsych Publications

CAMBRIDGE
UNIVERSITY PRESS

University Printing House, Cambridge CB2 8BS, United Kingdom

One Liberty Plaza, 20th Floor, New York, NY 10006, USA

477 Williamstown Road, Port Melbourne, VIC 3207, Australia

314-321, 3rd Floor, Plot 3, Splendor Forum, Jasola District Centre, New Delhi - 110025, India

79 Anson Road, #06-04/06, Singapore 079906

Cambridge University Press is part of the University of Cambridge.

It furthers the University's mission by disseminating knowledge in the pursuit of education, learning and research at the highest international levels of excellence.

www.cambridge.org
Information on this title: www.cambridge.org/9781904671534

© The Royal College of Psychiatrists 2007
Reprinted 2008, 2009, 2015

RCPsych Publications is an imprint of the Royal College of Psychiatrists, 21 Prescot Street, London E1 8BB
http://www.rcpsych.ac.uk

A catalogue record for this publication is available from the British Library

ISBN 978-1-904-67153-4 Paperback

Distributed in North America by Publishers Storage and Shipping Company.

Contents

Foreword

Stanley Smith Stevens defined measurement as 'the assignment of numbers to objects and events according to rules' (Stevens, 1951). This book provides an ideal starting point for researchers and clinicians in search of instruments with which to allocate 'numbers' in psychiatry.

There is a long an honourable tradition of measurement in psychiatry, since psychiatry has had to think much harder than other specialties about 'rules'. Psychiatry deals with concepts and phenomena that are important, but not as readily observable or measurable as in other clinical specialties. Notions of validity and reliability therefore need to be examined in some detail before a measurement instrument can be claimed to be a measurement of anything at all. Psychiatry's gift to the rest of medicine has been an appreciation of the importance of psychometrics and the development of some very good instruments. Historically, several instruments have found a place in wider medical practice (such as the Hospital Anxiety and Depression Scale). There are excellent instruments available for most areas of psychiatric practice, and clinicians and researchers are sometimes faced with a dizzying choice. Part of this choice stems from a 'measurement industry', whereby new instruments are continually developed and refined. Unfortunately, much of this happens without due consideration of what has gone before, and new is not necessarily better. In addition, some perfectly acceptable instruments are freely available in the public domain, whereas newer instruments sometimes come with an expensive price tag.

A little careful thought when choosing an instrument often saves time and money further down the line. There is a temptation to measure everything that is possible just because an instrument is available. The guiding principles when choosing outcome measures are to pick only those that measure what is important, and to choose instruments that are fit for purpose. Please bear in mind the effort involved in administering and filling in measurement instruments and always remember that 'less is more'. This book will help you in all these tasks.

Simon Gilbody

Stevens, S. (1951) Mathematics, measurement and psychophysics. In *Handbook of Experimental Psychology* (ed. S. Stevens), pp. 1–14. Wiley.

Introduction

Peter Tyrer and Caroline Methuen

Many years ago one of us (P.T.) was lecturing on the use of rating scales at a conference on research methodology. In a light-hearted way, the well-known acronym for the standard format of a rating scale, SPITZER, was introduced. 'Of course', went the explanation, 'we all know that the initials of the name stand for "Structured Psychiatric Interviews To Zealously Enhance Research", and the core of research methodology is to remember this, over and over again, when carrying out your research'. This explanation was a little too convincing because subsequently several people commented that they did not realise that Spitzer was only an acronym, not a real person, and it was an eye-opener to understand the real meaning of the word. We hasten to remind you that Robert Spitzer is a real person, who has added a great deal to the science of rating scales, and is mentioned several times in this booklet. One of Bob Spitzer's famous saws is, 'if it exists, it can be measured', and these seven words offer both a rationale and a strategy for using such scales. In this booklet we have unashamedly gone for a measure of esteem that many find intensely irritating, the citation rate, because we feel that the more a scale is cited the more value it is to the researcher, and particularly the systematic reviewer. Such a reviewer measuring temperature can accommodate the Fahrenheit and Celsius scales, but would be very put out if there were forty other scales also measuring temperature in completely different ways. By giving the citation rates (as of 2006) of each scale we are not necessarily saying the most cited one is the best, but, other things being equal, if most investigators chose a scale that is very widely used it would be much appreciated by the reviewer and ultimately by the researcher too. Nevertheless, the many-faceted presentations of psychiatry mean that often a standard scale is not appropriate for the subject matter and so a much less frequently cited scale would be better in a particular project. So the exposition of several scales is sometimes necessary in order to achieve the best fit, and very occasionally it may be necessary to construct your own scale for a specific piece of research: as we make very clear, this should be done only as a last resort.

So it only remains for you to look at the menu, ask the waiter and, if needed, the cook – don't be afraid to write to the author of the scale – to find out the exact nature of the fare, and then make your choice. *Bon appétit.*

Rating scales in psychiatry[†]

Peter Tyrer and Caroline Methuen

One of the most difficult tasks for aspiring research workers is choosing a rating scale. In an ideal world this should not be a difficult decision. Certain problems require special evaluation and, provided the problem has been recognised before, a suitable rating scale will exist for the purpose. If the rating scale is well established and is clearly the leader in the area, it will choose itself and there should be clear instructions on what training and expertise the researcher will need before the scale (or questionnaire) is applied. However, in practice choosing a rating scale is seldom this straightforward. This is mainly because there are too many rating scales and it is extremely difficult for the novice, and often even the expert, to choose the right scale easily. The rating scales described here are only a selection from a much larger pool; the abundance of new scales has made it impossible to cover the territory adequately. This booklet is therefore a general guide which should enable the researcher to identify the most appropriate scales for their area of interest, but a little more research will be required before the final choice of a scale is made. Hence we have given the main references for a large number of scales in the absence of space for an adequate review of each, on the premise that the wider the pool the better the eventual selection.

Choosing a rating scale

Figure 1 indicates the bumpy journey that the researcher will have to take before feeling confident that the right instrument has been chosen for the problem under investigation. The scales published in this booklet are by no means exhaustive so do not feel that it is unjustified for you to use a scale of your own choosing if you cannot find a measure for the subject under review in the pages below.

[†]This was first published as chapter 11 in Freeman, C. & Tyrer, P. (2006) *Research Methods in Psychiatry* (3rd edn). Gaskell.

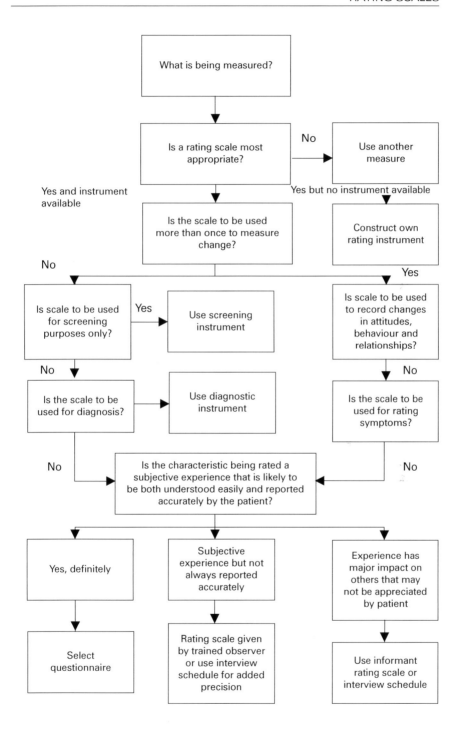

Fig. 1 Flow chart for selection of rating instruments in psychiatric research.

What is being measured?

Rating scales may not always be necessary in a study. As the use of rating scales involves administering an interview to an individual (patient or informant), the procedure is liable to natural attrition in any study, ranging from refusal to take part through to inability to follow-up. However, some other measures (e.g. admission to hospital) can be obtained from other sources and are more likely to yield complete data. There is also a strong and unnecessary tendency for junior researchers to collect as much data as possible without regard to its purpose. Investigators should elect at the design stage to ask whether every single item of information is essential, with the objective of eliminating at least half. The main advantage of simpler methods using few variables is that larger numbers of patients can often be accessed and so more robust findings are likely to emerge. It is therefore reasonable for the researcher to ask the question 'Can I get away without using a rating scale in this project?' It will save a tremendous amount of time and trouble if rating scales and questionnaires are avoided.

What is being measured and why?

There are three main uses for rating scales in psychiatry. The first is as a screening instrument which identifies a population with the condition of interest but could include some people without the condition. A screening instrument should have high sensitivity even though this may be achieved at the expense of low specificity.

The second reason for using a rating scale is to identify a feature that is felt to be important. Quite often this is a psychiatric diagnosis, but it could be any characteristic. The point of using the rating scale is to more accurately measure this characteristic and thereby improve the quality of the research, and also to compare the findings with other studies. First, for example, if one wanted to assess whether a specific personality disorder was associated with childhood physical abuse, the researcher might consider it necessary to assess such abuse (e.g. using the Child Trauma Questionnaire) rather than simply asking the patient a yes/no question.

The third reason for using an instrument is to record change, either spontaneously or following some type of intervention. This raises several other important questions. Is the instrument easy to administer, does repeated assessment lead to practice effects and is the administration of the instrument prone to bias of any sort?

The answer to these questions should determine the nature of the rating instrument selected and whether it is to be self-administered (i.e. a questionnaire) or administered by another person such as a researcher.

Source of information

Reliability always tends to increase with more structured scales and with trained interviewers. There is an understandable tendency to select such instruments (especially when trained interviewers are available) in order to improve the quality of the study, but, long before this, it needs to be asked who is providing the information and why. Thus, for example, if an intervention designed to reduce depression is being tested, it is appropriate to use a structured interview schedule of established reliability (e.g. Schedule for Affective Disorders and Schizophrenia; Endicott & Spitzer, 1978) for assessment, but if the person concerned has relatively mild symptoms that could be hidden from a stranger, it would be more appropriate to assess the patient with a self-rating scale (e.g. Hamilton Rating Scale for Depression; Hamilton, 1960).

Almost all psychiatric symptoms have both a subjective element and an objective one that is shown to others. In some instances there may be a gross disparity between the two (e.g. in the features of psychopathy), but it is rare to have one feature only. For this reason many investigators use both self-rating questionnaires and more 'objective' rating scales, although in practice these often show good levels of agreement.

One of the main advantages of the questionnaire is that it reduces the potential for bias because a patient is more likely to describe their own feelings accurately than an investigator who is involved in a comparison of treatments and has some knowledge of what these are. Often bias is unwitting and one advantage of recording both self-rated and observer-rated symptoms is that similar results with both types of instrument suggest a minimum of bias.

Devising your own instrument

Although there is a natural tendency for researchers to develop their own instruments on the premise that there is no scale available to measure a particular feature, this position is increasingly untenable as instruments become available for all aspects of psychiatric illness and treatments. There is also considerable concern that new and untested scales yield much larger effect sizes than well-established scales (i.e. overstate the difference between treatments; Marshall *et al*, 2000).

Although there are still circumstances when a new rating scale might be necessary for a specific project, it is important for researchers to be aware that such a scale should be evaluated and the results of the evaluation should be published before the scale is used in the planned study. This will invariably involve much more work than using an established scale. Nobody should believe that using a specially derived scale for a project is going to be a short cut to success.

In deciding on a new rating scale the investigator will have to make a distinction between a simple dichotomous scale, an interval scale and a visual analogue scale (Fig. 2). There is often a wish to modify an existing scale and although under some circumstances this is justifiable, it must not be done without a great deal of thought, as comparisons with data using the original scale would thereby be rendered invalid.

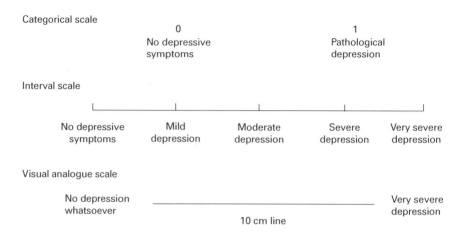

Fig. 2 Examples of types of rating scale: categorical scale, interval scale (implying dimensions, e.g. Likert scale) and visual analogue scale (the participant is asked to place a vertical mark across the line at the point that best describes current feelings; this is measured to give a 'depression score').

Finding a rating scale

The rest of this booklet lists the main scales for each area of psychiatry. This is a repetitive exercise but it is clear from talking to novice researchers that the listing of these scales is important. We decided that the main criterion for the inclusion a scale should be the extent of its use (as the wider the use of a scale the better will be comparability with other studies). We have therefore calculated the citation rate per year of each scale since the year of publication and only those scales that are widely cited in the literature (with a cut-off point of 4.0 per year for general scales and 2.0 per year for specific ones) have been included. Although we are well aware that some of the most commonly used scales are not quite as good as some others and have only achieved their status by a combination of primacy, luck and salesmanship, their frequency of use is still the best single criterion for the research worker in making a choice. Where the details of scales are not available in the published references the researcher is advised to search for these on the internet. This is now much easier with improved search engines such as Google, and any scale which is searched for using the author's name and title of the scale should be found easily. The most popular scales are frequently copyrighted and distributed by commercial publishers. For those that are less widely used but seem to be appropriate for a study it does no harm to get in touch with the originator(s). They will be flattered (unless of course the scale is so widely used it has led to many previous enquiries) and may offer extra help in starting the project. This may even be worthwhile

Table 1   Rating scales and questionnaires for depression

Author(s)	Type of assessment	Citation rate per year and comments
Hamilton (1960)	Hamilton Rating Scale for Depression (HRSD)	199.5 (the original and, to many, still the best)
Beck et al (1961)	Beck Depression Inventory (BDI)	186.2 (competing for the crown with enthusiasm – generally preferred in more recent studies)
Zigmond & Snaith (1983)	Hospital Anxiety and Depression Scale (HAD)	133.0 (currently the most frequently used self-rating scale, equally good for anxiety)
Montgomery & Åsberg (1979)	Montgomery–Åsberg Depression Rating Scale (MADRS)	83.2 (derived from the Comprehensive Psychopathological Rating Scale (CPRS) and may be of special value when multiple pathology is being assessed; very often used in short-term studies of interventions, particularly drugs)
Zung (1965)	Zung Self-Rating Depression Scale	78.9 (the original self-rating scale; still widely used)
Brink et al (1982)	Geriatric Depression Scale (GDS)	71.9 (clear preference for this scale in studies of older adults)
Beck et al (1974b)	Hopelessness Scale	38.9 (very frequently used in studies of suicide)
Cox et al (1987)	Edinburgh Postnatal Depression Scale (EPDS)	33.1 (the established scale for assessing depression in relationship to childbirth) Also see Cox & Holden (2003)
Seligman et al (1979)	Attributional Style Questionnaire	22.4
Alexopoulus et al (1988)	Cornell Scale for Depression in Dementia	22 (an example of a special area in which a general scale may not be accurate)
Carney et al (1965)	ECT Scale (Newcastle)	21.4 (was once very widely used but less so recently, as the distinction between depressive syndromes is less often required)
Kandel & Davies (1982)	Six-Item Depression Mood Inventory	15.4
Brown & Harris (1978)	Life Events and Difficulties Scale (LEDS)	11.2 (the definitive life events assessment scale – needs prior training – listed here as the work was primarily concerned with depression)
Zuckerman (1960)	Multiple Affect Adjective Checklist (MAACL)	8.5. (checklists used to be very common methods of assessing mood states but are now less often used)

continued

Table 1 *continued*

Author(s)	Type of assessment	Citation rate per year and comments
Robinson *et al* (1993)	Pathological Laughter and Crying Scale	8.2
Raskin *et al* (1969)	Raskin Three-Area Depression Rating Scale	7.9
McNair & Lorr (1964)	Profile of Mood States (POMS)	7.63 (a very widely used simple scale, but not used so much in recent years)
Snaith *et al* (1971)	Wakefield Self-Assessment Depression Inventory	6.97 (now replaced mainly by Hospital Anxiety and Depression Scale)
Steiner *et al* (1980)	Premenstrual Tension Syndrome Scale (PMTS)	6.8
Snaith *et al* (1976)	Leeds Scales for the Self-Assessment of Anxiety and Depression	6.71 (as for Wakefield Scale)
Lubin (1965)	Depression Adjective Check-List (DACL)	6.3
Sunderland *et al* (1988)	Dementia Mood Assessment Scale	5.6
Costello & Comfrey (1967)	Costello's Scales for Measuring Depression and Anxiety	5
Berrios *et al* (1992)	Guilt Scale	3.9

Table 2 Rating scales for mania

Author(s)	Type of assessment	Citation rate per year and comments
Young *et al* (1978)	Young Mania Rating Scale	21.5 (a short scale now well established in research studies of all kinds and the clear leader)
Bech *et al* (1986)	Bech–Rafaelsen Rating Scale for Mania	3.6 (particularly useful when severe depression (melancholia) also being measured, as Bech–Rafaelsen Rating Scale for Melancholia can also be used)
Altman *et al* (1994)	Clinician-Administered Rating Scale for Mania (CARS–M)	3.5 (good psychometric properties but not widely used)

with the more established scales, and can sometimes lead to a great deal of extra help in both using and analysing results.

Depression and mania

Depression (next to anxiety) is probably the most common psychiatric symptom and so there are many scales for its measurement. However, only five (Table 1) are used frequently in current research studies and the choice is not as difficult as might have been expected. In contrast, mania is less common and there are considerably fewer scales, of which the Young Mania Rating Scale is the most often chosen (Table 2). For studies in which both mania and depression are investigated the Bech–Rafaelsen scales for both mania and melancholia (Bech et al, 1986) may be most appropriate. As depression can occur in so many different clinical contexts there is scope for many other instruments for its measurement. The Edinburgh Postnatal Depression Scale (Cox et al, 1987) (Table 1) is probably the best example of a more specialised scale, but all of the specialised scales closely correlate with the general scales and have overlapping questions.

Cognitive function and impairment (including assessments specific to old age)

Although mood disturbance may be the most common psychiatric symptom, cognitive function, in its many forms, is probably most frequently assessed. It is now accepted that something more than clinical questioning is needed to assess cognitive functioning and this is demonstrated by the success of the Mini Mental State Examination (MMSE; Table 3) and its modified form (3MS; Teng & Chui, 1987) as part of clinical assessment (Aquilina & Warner, 2004). The ordinary assessment of mental state is being supplemented by a more formal measure that can be scored and helps to quantify any impairment. As the average age of the population increases, so will the use of these scales.

Eating disorders

The symptomatology and related clinical features of eating disorders show important differences from other syndromes in psychiatry and require assessment with appropriate specialised scales. Although self-rating scales are commonly used, there is a problem with their validity at some stages of illness, particularly in severe anorexia when patients often deny obvious symptomatology (Halmi, 1985). The two most frequently used scales are the Eating Attitudes Test (Garner & Garfinkel, 1979) and the Eating Attitudes Inventory (Garner et al, 1983), but bulimia is often assessed using different scales (Halmi et al, 1981; Henderson & Freeman, 1987) (Table 4). However, no one scale achieves clear primacy in this area.

Table 3 Scales for assessment of cognitive function and old age symptomatology

Author(s)	Name of scale	Citations per year and comments
Folstein *et al* (1975)	Mini Mental State Examination (MMSE)	528.9 (The ultimate success of a rating scale is to be incorporated into standard clinical practice. The MMSE has now achieved this status – at least for the time being.)
Hughes *et al* (1982)	Clinical Dementia Rating (CDR)	68.1
Hachinski *et al* (1975)	Ischemia Score	66.1
Blessed *et al* (1968)	Blessed Dementia Rating Scale (BDRS) Information – Memory – Concentration Test (IMCT)	62.7
Gottfries *et al* (1982*a,b*)	Gottfries–Brane–Steen Dementia Rating Scale (GBS)	61
Reisberg *et al* (1982)	Global Deterioration Scale (GDS)	55.7
Katz *et al* (1963)	Index of Activities of Daily Living	52.7 (included here as this assessment is so often linked to cognitive assessment but could also be included under social function)
Cummings *et al* (1994)	Neuropsychiatric Inventory (NPI)	50.4
Mohs *et al* (1983)	Alzheimer's Disease Assessment Scale (ADAS)	42.5
Lawton & Brody (1969); Lawton (1988*a,b*)	Instrumental Activities of Daily Living (IADL) Scale	41.3 (as for Katz *et al* 1963)
Pfeiffer (1975)	Short Portable Mental Status Questionnaire (SPMSQ)	41.2
Plutchik *et al* (1970)	Geriatric Rating Scale (GRS)	34
Teng & Chui (1987)	Modified Mini-Mental State (3MS) Examination	26.7
Neugarten *et al* (1961)	Life Satisfaction Index (LSI)	19.5
Roth *et al* (1988)	Cambridge Mental Disorders of the Elderly Examination (CAMDEX)	17.7 (increasingly being used in non-US studies)
Katzman *et al* (1983)	Orientation–Memory–Concentration Test (OMCT)	17
Broadbent *et al* (1982)	Cognitive Failures Questionnaire (CFQ)	16.8
Lawton *et al* (1982)	Multilevel Assessment Instrument (MAI)	16.5

continued

Table 3 *continued*

Author(s)	Name of scale	Citations per year and comments
Copeland *et al* (1976)	Geriatric Mental State Schedule (GMS)	15.8
Copeland *et al* (1986)	Geriatric Mental State Schedule and Diagnostic Schedule (AGECAT)	15.7
Teri *et al* (1992)	Revised memory and behaviour checklist	14.8
Hodkinson (1972)	Mental Test Score	14.3
Lawton (1975)	Philadelphia Geriatric Center Morale Scale	13.9
Wells (1979)	Checklist Differentiating Pseudo-Dementia from Dementia	13.7
Gelinas & Gauthier (1999)	Disability Assessment for Dementia (DAD)	12.6
Inouye *et al* (1990)	Confusion assessment method (CAM)	11.9
Greene *et al* (1982)	Relative's Stress Scale	10.1
Greene *et al* (1982)	Behaviour and Mood Disturbance Scale	10
Knopman *et al* (1994)	Clinicians Interview-Based Impression (CIBI)	10
Soloman *et al* (1998)	Seven minute neurocognitive screening battery	9.8
Pattie & Gilleard (1979)	Clifton Assessment Procedures for the Elderly (CAPE)	9.6
Reisberg (1988)	Functional Assessment Staging (FAST)	9.6
Trzepacz *et al* (1988)	Delirium Rating Scale (DRS)	9.3
Jorm & Jacomb (1989)	Informant Questionnaire on Cognitive Decline in the Elderly (IQCODE)	9.3
Shader *et al* (1974)	Sandoz Clinical Assessment–Geriatric (SCAG) Scale	8.2
Cohen-Mansfield *et al* (1989)	Cohen-Mansfield Agitation Inventory (CMAI)	8.1
Kopelman *et al* (1990)	Autobiographical Memory Interview (AMI)	7.4

continued

11

Table 3 *continued*

Author(s)	Name of scale	Citations per year and comments
Gurland *et al* (1976, 1977)	Comprehensive Assessment and Referral Evaluation (CARE)	6.7
Logsdon & Gibbons (1999)	Quality of Life in Alzheimer's Disease (QoL–AD)	6.6
Hall *et al* (1993)	Bilingual Dementia Screening Interview	5.6
Reisberg & Ferris (1988)	Brief Cognitive Rating Scale (BCRS)	4.7
Spiegel *et al* (1991)	Nurses' Observation Scale for Geriatric Patients (NOSGER)	4.6
Hope & Fairburn (1992)	Present Behavioural Examination (PBE)	4.6
Patel & Hope (1992)	Rating Scale for Aggressive Behaviour in the Elderly – The RAGE	4.5
Wilkinson & Graham-White (1980)	Edinburgh Psychogeriatric Dependency Rating Scale (PGDRS)	4.5
Jorm *et al* (1995)	Psychogeriatric Assessment Scales (PAS)	4.2
Allen *et al* (1996)	Manchester and Oxford Universities Scale for the Psychopathological Assessment of Dementia (MOUSEPAD)	4 (close to getting an award for the most inventive acronym for a scale)
Qureshi & Hodkinson (1974)	Abbreviated Mental Test (AMT)	4
Helmes *et al* (1987)	Multidimensional Observation Scale for Elderly Subjects (MOSES)	3.6
Adshead *et al* (1992)	Brief Assessment Schedule Depression Cards (BASDEC)	3.4 (simple assessment using cards in similar situations to those for Cornell Scale for Depression in Dementia)
Sclan & Saillon (1996)	BEHAVE–AD	3.1
Kendrick *et al* (1979)	Kendrick Battery for the Detection of Dementia in the Elderly	2.8
Meer & Baker (1966)	Stockton Geriatric Rating Scale (SGRS)	2.7
Kuriansky & Gurland (1976)	Performance Test of Activities of Daily Living (PADL)	2.6
Bucks *et al* (1996)	Bristol Activities of Daily Living Scale	2.6
Schwartz (1983)	Geriatric Evaluation by Relative's Rating Instrument (GERRI)	2.5
Hersch (1979)	Extended Scale for Dementia (ESD)	2.3

Table 4 Instruments for the measurement of symptoms and attitudes in eating disorders

Author(s)	Name of scale	Citations per year and comments
Garner *et al* (1983)	Body Dissatisfaction Subscale of the Eating Disorder Inventory (EDI)	56.7 (The EDI is the most commonly used measure with a range of sub-scales – better for anorexia than bulimia)
Stunkard & Messick (1985)	Eating Inventory	42.1
Garner & Garfinkel (1979)	Eating Attitudes Test (EAT)	40.8
Halmi *et al* (1981)	Binge Eating Questionnaire	22
Cooper *et al* (1987)	Body Shape Questionnaire	16.5
Van Strien *et al* (1986)	Dutch Eating Behaviour Questionnaire (DEBQ)	16.1
Cooper & Fairburn (1987)	Eating Disorders Examination (EDE)	15.9 (semi-structured interview covering both bulimia and anorexia)
Morgan & Russell (1975)	Morgan–Russell Assessment Schedule (MRAS)	15.9 (often used in long-term outcome studies)
Gormally *et al* (1982)	Binge Eating Scale	12.7
Henderson & Freeman (1987)	Bulimic Investigatory Test, Edinburgh (BITE)	12.2 (short (33-item) questionnaire suitable for surveys)
Hawkins & Clement (1980)	Binge Scale	11.8
Smith & Thelen (1984)	Bulimia Test (BULIT)	8.6
Slade & Russell (1973)	Anorexic Behaviour Scale (ABS)	7.0
Johnson (1985)	Diagnostic Survey for Eating Disorders (DSED)	5.5
Slade *et al* (1990)	Body Satisfaction Scale (BSS)	3.1
Fichter *et al* (1989)	Structured Interview for anorexia and Bulimia Nervosa (SIAB)	3
Ben-Tovim & Walker (1991)	Ben-Tovim Walker Body Attitudes Questionnaire (BAQ)	2.9
Slade & Dewey (1986)	Setting Conditions for Anorexia Nervosa (SCANS)	2.3

General functioning and symptomatology

Psychiatry as a discipline used to be criticised because it did not use the language of science and measurement and so could be interpreted in so many different ways. The discipline responded (some might say overreacted) to this criticism by introducing a much more rigid and reliable set of diagnoses, the *Diagnostic and Statistical Manual for Mental Disorders* (3rd edn) (DSM–III) (American Psychiatric Association, 1980). By introducing operational criteria for the definition of each diagnosis a much greater level of reliability was achieved, but it is well known that improvements in reliability are often achieved at the expense of validity. This was a central issue of the life work of Robert Kendell (1925–2002), who pointed out that the only valid diagnosis was the one that demonstrated a 'point of rarity' between it and other diagnoses, in the same way that many organic diagnoses do in medicine. In fact, almost every psychiatric diagnosis is best perceived as a continuum or dimension rather than a separate and discrete category. This is not a criticism of the diagnostic process, since the identification of a psychiatric diagnosis may still be extremely useful in clinical practice; what must not be assumed is that clinical utility is the same as clinical validity (Kendell & Jablensky, 2003). This basic understanding of psychiatric diagnoses as a continuum is one of the reasons why scales measuring general functioning and symptomatology are becoming more popular; they are recording the dimensions.

Researchers will also wish to measure global psychopathology when the population being studied is a heterogeneous one in which all aspects of symptomatology need to be detected. Epidemiological studies of whole populations and cohort studies that examine change and new pathology over time are the most common examples. Many of the scales are linked to diagnoses, particularly DSM ones, and this probably explains why the SCID group (Structured Clinical Interviews for DSM Diagnoses) are so popular (Table 5). However, research workers should note that DSM–V is going to be very different from its predecessors and it is wise not to be too attached to measurement scales that are related to a changing system.

Satisfaction and needs

There is now a realisation of the importance of the consumer in mental health services, and although the word 'user' is not entirely satisfactory, the balance of influence is gradually shifting towards those who receive treatment from those who do the treating. We therefore have a range of relatively new instruments to measure need and satisfaction with services that are now becoming *de rigeur* in many research arenas. The best known of these is probably the Camberwell Assessment of Need (CAN; Phelan

Table 5 Scales for general functioning and symptomatology

Author(s)	Name of scale	Citations per year and comments
Spitzer *et al* (1990*a,b, d*)	Structured Clinical Interview for DSM–III–R (SCID)	165.6 (simple and straightforward scales that lack some subtlety but are widely used because of their DSM links)
Spitzer *et al* (1990*c*)	Structured Clinical Interview for DSM–III–R personality disorders (SCID–II)	162.7
Robins *et al* (1981)	Diagnostic Interview Schedule (DIS)	135.1
Wing *et al* (1974)	Present State Examination and Catego Program (PSE)	112.4 (now being replaced by SCAN, which incorporates much of the old PSE)
Endicott *et al* (1976)	Global Assessment Scale (GAS), later to become Global Assessment of Functioning (GAF)	76.3 (a scale that is now an axis of pathology – Axis 5 in the DSM classification) (may be separated into symptomatology and functioning components)
Goldberg (1972)	General Health Questionnaire (GHQ)	59.0 (the doyen of quick screening for common mental disorders)
Scheier & Carver (1985)	Life Orientation Test (LOT)	53.6
Derogatis *et al* (1973)	Symptom Check-List (SCL-90)	50.8 (very popular quick assessment of psychopathology but coming to the end of its useful life)
Derogatis *et al* (1974)	Hopkins Symptom Checklist (HSCL)	45.2 (linked to SCL-90)
Robins *et al* (1988)	The Composite International Diagnostic Interview (CIDI)	44.0 (rapidly becoming the benchmark for national epidemiological studies (except in the UK, where CIS–R is still used)
Åsberg *et al* (1978)	Comprehensive Psychopathological Rating Scale (CPRS)	33 (has the advantage of being linked to sub-scales for depression, anxiety, and obsessional and schizophrenic pathology)
Wing *et al* (1990)	SCAN – Schedules for Clinical Assessment in Neuropsychiatry	30.9 (the successor to the PSE, shortly to come out in a revised form (SCAN–II))
McGuffin *et al* (1991)	Operational criteria for psychotic illnesses	28.5 (useful when information needs to be obtained from notes and other records – may be converted to several diagnostic systems)
Millon (1981)	Millon Clinical Multiaxial Inventory (MCMI)	27 (a very popular personality assessment even though it does not match with DSM or ICD)

continued

Table 5 *continued*

Author(s)	Name of scale	Citations per year and comments
Goldberg *et al* (1970)	Clinical Interview Schedule (CIS)	20.4 (see also CIS–R)
Aitken (1969)	Visual Analogue Scales	20.1 (these are often useful when making self-ratings or in contructing one's own scales)
Dupuy (1984)	Psychological General Well-Being (PGWB) Index	19
Lewis *et al* (1992)	Clinical Interview Schedule – Revised (CIS–R)	17.8 (a scale specially developed for epidemiological studies with lay interviewers – has now mainly replaced the CIS)
Raskin & Crook (1988)	Relative's Assessment of Global Symptomatology (RAGS)	7
Spitzer *et al* (1970)	Psychiatric Status Schedule (PSS)	6.7
Brodman *et al* (1949)	Cornell Medical Index	6.6
Spanier (1987)	Dyadic Adjustment Scale	5.4
Luborsky (1962)	Health Sickness Rating Scale (HSRS)	5.3 (the forerunner of the GAF)
Burnam *et al* (1983)	Spanish Diagnostic Interview Schedule	5.1
Helzer & Robins (1981)	Renard Diagnostic Interview	4.8
Endicott & Spitzer (1972)	Current and Past Psychopathology Scales (CAPPS)	4.7
Marmar *et al* (1986)	California Psychotherapy Alliances Scales (CALPAS–T/P)	3.8
Power *et al* (1988)	Significant Others Scale (SOS)	3.8
Parloff *et al* (1954)	Symptom Check-List (SCL)	3.6
Lorr *et al* (1962)	Lorr's Multidimensional Scale for Rating Psychiatric Patients	2.3
Spitzer *et al* (1967)	Mental Status Schedule (MSS)	2.3

Table 6 Scales for the assessment of need and satisfaction

Author(s)	Name of scale	Citations per year and comments
Phelan *et al* (1995)	Camberwell Assessment of Need (CAN); CANE (Elderly), CANDID (Intellectual Disability), CANFOR (Forensic Psychiatry), CANSAS (Short Appraisal Schedule)	16.1 (now the most widely used scale in the area; the sub-scales have yet to be widely used)
Beecher (1959)	Measurement of Subjective Responses (MSR)	15.1 (useful in assessing the placebo effect)
Larsen *et al* (1979)	Consumer Satisfaction Questionnaire (CSQ)	14.5 (is rapidly becoming the most commonly used scale for measuring general satisfaction)
Amador *et al* (1993)	Scale to Assess Unawareness of Mental Disorder	13.1
Harding *et al* (1980)	Self Report Questionnaire (SRQ)	11.7
Bech (1993)	Psychological General Well-Being Schedule (PGWBS)	11.4
Bunney & Hamburg (1963)	Bunney–Hamburg Mood Check-list	10.8
Brewin *et al* (1987)	MRC Needs for Care Assessment	7.9 (the predecessor to CAN and probably its catalyst)
Ruggeri & Dall'Agnola (1993)	Verona Service Satisfaction Scale (VSSS)	6.2 (specifically developed for measuring satisfaction with mental health services)
Birchwood *et al* (1994)	Insight Scale (for Psychosis)	6.1 (the measurement of insight is becoming increasingly important in research studies)
Markova & Berrios (1992)	Insight Scale	3.8
Shipley *et al* (2000)	Patient Satisfaction Questionnaire	2.3
Tantam (1988)	The Express Scale and Personality Questionnaire	2.3

et al, 1995) and its many successors (CANSAS, CANFOR, CANDID, etc.), the latest being CAN–M for mothers. However, there are many others that attempt to assess patients' experiences and feelings towards their condition and treatment in a variety of settings (Table 6).

Self-harm

Self-harm has come to replace the earlier term 'parasuicide' and the misleading one 'attempted suicide' as a description of the behaviour of those who do not usually carry out their acts of harm with the intention of killing themselves, but who might do so by accident and are at much greater risk of successful suicide in the future (Jenkins *et al*, 2002; Zahl & Hawton, 2004). The chances of repeat attempts and successful suicide are greater when suicidal intent is greater (Zahl & Hawton, 2004) and so measures of this and other elements of risk are useful) (Table 7). There is evidence that such scales are successful in predicting self-harm (Tyrer *et al*, 2003).

Sexual behaviour

Although sexual behaviour has rarely been measured systematically in many psychiatric studies when it is clearly relevant (e.g. in patients with schizophrenia on antipsychotic drugs), such measurement is now

Table 7   Scales for the assessment of self-harm

Author(s)	Name of scale	Citations per year
Beck *et al* (1974*a*)	Beck Hopelessness Scale	43.7[1]
Beck *et al* (1979)	Scale for Suicide Ideation (SSI)	12.7
Beck *et al* (1974*b*)	Suicidal Intent Scale (SIS)	12
Motto *et al* (1985)	Risk Estimator for Suicide	4.2
Pallis *et al* (1982)	Post-Attempt Risk Assessment Scale	2.6
Plutchik *et al* (1989)	Suicide Risk Scale (SRS)	2.5
Buglass & Horton (1974)	Risk of Repetition Scale	2.3
Tuckman & Youngman (1968)	Scale for Assessing Suicide Risk of Attempted Suicides	2.3
Kreitman & Foster (1991)	Parasuicide Risk Scale	2.3

1. By far the most quoted and used scale, although hopelessness not strictly a self-harm measure.

becoming both more accepted and acceptable in research studies. For this reason a greater number of scales is given in Table 8 than is strictly necessary as their citation rate has been fairly low.

Substance use, dependence and withdrawal

The assessment of substance misuse is prone to error, mainly because the reliability of the information is often so uncertain. Hence there is an increasing tendency to use modern techniques such as hair analysis to obtain independent evidence of drug use. Table 9 includes some scales that are becoming established assessments for research studies; AUDIT, MAST, CAGE and SDS are the most frequently used. Most scales in Table 9 are concerned with dependence.

Increasingly it is becoming necessary to record symptoms of withdrawal following the cessation of illicit or prescribed drugs. Because each group of substances has different withdrawal effects (in addition to many common ones) it is probably preferable to select a scale to suit the substance (Table 10) rather than use a general scale.

Personality assessment and persistent behaviours

Personality assessment is one of the more difficult subjects to tackle in research. Like IQ, we like to think of personality as stable, but empirical studies have shown it is much less stable than we would like to think. However, when assessing personality we are not just assessing present

Table 8   Scales for the assessment of sexual function and behaviour

Author(s)	Name of scale	Citations per year
Lopiccolo & Steger (1974)	Sexual Interaction Inventory	50
Wilhelm & Parker (1988)	Intimate Bond Measure (IBM)	4
Hoon *et al* (1976)	Sexual Arousal Inventory (SAI)	3.9
Nichols & Molinder (1984)	Multiphasic Sex Inventory (MSI)	2.8
Eysenck (1971)	Eysenck Inventory of Attitudes to Sex	1.9
Golombok & Rust (1985)	Golombok–Rust Inventory of Sexual Satisfaction (GRISS)	1.6
Derogatis (1978)	Derogatis Sexual Functioning Inventory (DSFI)	1.3
Frenken & Vennix (1981)	Sexual Experience Scales (SES)	1.2

Table 9 Scales for the assessment of substance use and dependence

Author(s)	Name of scale	Citations per year and comments
Saunders *et al* (1993)	Alcohol Use Disorders Identification Test (AUDIT)	45.3 (used for the identification of hazardous and harmful alcohol consumption)
Selzer (1971)	Michigan Alcoholism Screening Test (MAST)	42.1
Mayfield *et al* (1974)	CAGE Questionnaire	27.6
Gossop *et al* (1995)	The Severity of Dependence Scale (SDS)	13.8 (used in heroin, amphetamine and cocaine dependence)
McLennan *et al* (1980)	Addiction Severity Index	5
Skinner & Allen (1983)	Alcohol Dependence Scale (ADS)	2.8
Chick (1980)	Edinburgh Alcohol Dependence Scale	2.3
Halikas *et al* (1991)	Minnesota Cocaine Craving Scale	2.2
Smith *et al* (1996)	Paddington Alcohol Test (PAT)	2.1 (used to detect hazardous drinking in patients presenting as emergencies)
Horn *et al* (1974)	Alcohol Use Inventory	2.1
Litman *et al* (1983)	Coping Behaviour Inventory (CBI)	2
Litman *et al* (1984)	Effectiveness of Coping Behaviour Inventory (ECBI)	1.9
Washton *et al* (1988)	Cocaine Abuse Assessment Profile (CAAP)	1.1
Skinner & Goldberg (1986)	Drug Abuse Screening Test (DAST)	1.1

Table 10 Scales for the assessment of substance use withdrawal problems

Author(s)	Name of scale	Citations per year
Chaney *et al* (1978)	Situational Competency Test (SCT)	8.7
Gross *et al* (1973)	TSA and SSA	5.9
Raistrick *et al* (1983)	Short Alcohol Dependence Data (SADD)	4.4
Tyrer *et al* (1990)	Benzodiazepine Withdrawal Symptom Questionnaire	4.2
Handelsman *et al* (1987)	Objective Opiate Withdrawal Scale (OOWS)	3.5
Handelsman *et al* (1987)	Subjective Opiate Withdrawal Scale	3.5
Annis (1986)	Situational Confidence Questionnaire	2.7
Sutherland *et al* (1986)	Severity of Opiate Dependence Questionnaire (SODQ)/Opiate Subjective Dependence Questionnaire (OSDQ)	2.4

personality function but characteristic function over a long period. This cannot be done easily but there are many attempts to shorten the assessment process in order to fit in with the multiple assessments being performed over a short time period. Most assessments are carried out using the DSM recommendations for personality disorders, even though these are now recognised to be grossly unsatisfactory and redundant in research terms (Livesley, 2001). Persistent behavioural problems such as aggression are also included in Table 11. There is also a very important group of instruments that measure risk of violence and these are becoming more commonly used in research studies as their predictive quality improves. The Psychopathy Checklist–Revised (PCL–R; Hare, 1991) is the best known but there are also many others (Dolan & Doyle, 2000).

Anxiety and associated disorders

Anxiety is ubiquitous, easy to measure but difficult to interpret. There has been much argument over the differences between state and trait anxiety and their significance, the meaning of the association of anxiety and depression (the two are intimate) and the importance of anxiety to the course and development of phobic, obsessional, hypochondriacal, pain, post-traumatic and fatigue disorders. These subjects are therefore included in Tables 12 and 13.

Sleep

Despite being somewhat relegated to the sidelines of psychiatry in recent years, sleep problems remain very prominent symptoms of mental illness. It is always possible to assess sleep problems from individual items in scales for depression and anxiety but for general sleep satisfaction and performance it is preferable to use one of the scales in Table 14.

Schizophrenia and related psychotic disorders

Although there continues to be debate over the issues of insight, adherence to therapy and the relationship between schizotypy and schizophrenia, the core assessment of schizophrenic pathology involves assessment with relatively few instruments, of which the Schedule for Affective Disorders and Schizophrenia (SADS) and Scales for the Assessment of Positive and Negative Symptoms (SAPS and SANS) are the most popular, and are gradually replacing the Brief Psychiatric Rating Scale (BPRS; Overall & Gorham, 1962) from the lead position it has held for most of the past 40 years (Table 15). The major change has been in the recognition of positive and negative symptoms and the need to record them separately. The different therapeutic profile of drugs such as clozapine has helped in this

Table 11   Scales for assessing personality and persistent behavioural problems

Authors	Name of scale	Citations per year and comments
Spitzer *et al* (1990*c*)	Structured Clinical Interview for DSM–III–R Personality Disorders (SCID–II)	162.7
Buss & Durkee (1957)	Buss–Durkee Hostility and Guild Inventory	23.6
Spielberger *et al* (1985)	State–Trait Anger Expression Inventory (STAXI)	23.2
Pfohl *et al* (1983)	Structured Interview for DSM–III Personality Disorders (SID–P)	17.9
Yudofsky (1986)	Overt Aggression Scale (OAS)	17.3 (may also be used in modified form as the Modified Overt Aggression Scale (MOAS) (Sorgi *et al*, 1991))
Hathaway & McKinley (1967)	Minnesota Multiphasic Personality Inventory (MMPI)	16.6
Gunderson *et al* (1981)	Diagnostic Interview for Borderline Patients	15.6
Loranger *et al* (1985)	Personality Disorder Examination (PDE)	14
Tyrer & Alexander (1979)	Personality Assessment Schedule (PAS)	13.8
Rosenbaum (1980)	Self Control Schedule	13.2
Barron (1953)	Barron Ego Strength	10.9
Hare (1980)	Psychopathy Checklist (PCL)	10.2 (the best predictor of aggressive behaviour in psychiatric patients (Monahan *et al*, 2001); was revised in 1990 (PCL–R) and again in 2004; special training is required which is unlikely to be possible within the budget of simple research projects)
Hyler & Reider (1987)	Personality Diagnostic Questionnaire – Revised (PDQ–R)	9.8
Morey *et al* (1985)	Modified Minnesota Multiphasic Personality Inventory (MMPI)	9.1

continued

Table 11 *continued*

Authors	Name of scale	Citations per year and comments
Schwartz & Gottman (1976)	Assertiveness Self-Statement Test (ASST)	6.3
Glass *et al* (1982)	Social Interaction Self-Statement Test (SISST)	6.2
Palmstierna & Wistedt (1987)	Staff Observation and Aggression Scale (SOAS)	5.8
Baron *et al* (1981)	Schedule for Interviewing Schizotypal Personalities (SSP)	5.2
Conte *et al* (1980)	Borderline Syndrome Index (BSI)	5
Robson (1989)	Robson's Self-Esteem Scale	4.3
Bell (1981)	Bell Object Relations Self-Report Scale	3.8
Mann *et al* (1981)	Standardized Assessment of Personality (SAP)	3.7
Hyler *et al* (1982)	Personality Diagnostic Questionnaire (PDQ)	3.5
Galissi *et al* (1981)	Checklist of Positive and Negative Thoughts	3.2
Lorr & Youniss (1983)	Interpersonal Style Inventory (ISI)	2.1

Table 12 Scales for hypochondriasis, health anxiety, pain and fatigue

Author(s)	Name of scale	Citations per year
Fukuda *et al* (1994)	Chronic Fatigue Syndrome – case-defining symptoms	87.4 (important for examining chronic fatigue and formalising description of cases)
Melzack (1987)	McGill Pain Questionnaire (MPQ)	29.6
Chalder *et al* (1993)	Fatigue Scale	22.6
Pilowsky & Spence (1975)	Illness Behaviour Questionnaire (IBQ)	7.4
Kellner (1987)	Symptom questionnaire	7.2 (now mainly of historical interest)
Barsky *et al* (1990)	Somatosensory Amplification Scale (SSAS)	7.1 (may be useful to detect health anxiety)
Salkovskis *et al* (2002)	Health Anxiety Inventory (HAI)	2.3 (specifically used for health anxiety, which is not quite the same as the old concept of hypochondriasis)

Table 13 Scales for assessment of anxiety and related symptoms

Authors	Name of scale	Citations per year and comments
Zigmond & Snaith (1983)	Hospital Anxiety and Depression Scale (HADS)	133.0 (the anxiety version (HADS–A) can also be combined with the depression component (HADS–D) to score mixed anxiety–depressive symptoms (cothymia) (Tyrer, 2001))
Spielberger *et al* (1983)	Spielberger State–Trait Anxiety Inventory (STAI)	121.4 (commonly used in repeated measures studies – in which both present state and trait anxiety are measured separately)
Goodman *et al* (1989*a,b*)	Yale–Brown Obsessive Compulsive Scale (Y–BOCS)	81.1 (the standard scale for measurement of obsessive–compulsive symptoms – clearly now pre-eminent)
Beck *et al* (1988)	Beck Anxiety Inventory (BAI)	49.8 (beginning to usurp the Hamilton scale)
Hamilton (1959)	Hamilton Anxiety Scale (HAS)	45.6 (an observer-rated scale that remains standard but has been criticised for its emphasis on somatic symptoms that may reflect physical illness)
Taylor (1953)	Taylor Manifest Anxiety Scale (TMAS)	44.4 (really a measure of trait anxiety)
Marks & Mathews (1979)	Brief Standard Self-Rating Scale for Phobic Patients	36.2 (the most common self-rating for common phobic symptoms)
Keane *et al* (1988)	Mississippi Scale for Combat-Related Post-traumatic Stress Disorder	35.8
Watson & Friend (1969)	Fear of Negative Evaluation Scale (FNE)	28.3
Watson & Friend (1969)	Social Avoidance and Distress Scale (SAD)	28.3
Chambless *et al* (1984)	Body Sensations Questionnaire and the Agoraphobic Cognitions Questionnaire	20
Chambless *et al* (1985)	Mobility Inventory for Agoraphobia	18.8
Wolpe & Lang (1964)	Fear Survey Schedule (FSS)	14.9
Zung (1971)	Zung's Anxiety Status Inventory (ASI)	13.6
Alderman *et al* (1983)	Crown-Crisp Experiential Index (CCEI)	13.1
Hodgson & Rachman (1977)	Maudsley Obsessional-Compulsive Inventory	13.1

continued

Table 13 *continued*

Authors	Name of scale	Citations per year and comments
Beck *et al* (1987)	Cognitions Checklist–Anxiety (CCL–A)	10.8 (relevant in monitoring cognitive–behavioural therapy)
Davidson *et al* (1997)	Davidson Trauma Scale (DTS)	10.6
Cooper (1970)	Leyton Obsessional Inventory	9.6
Sanavio (1988)	Padua Inventory	8.3
Steinberg *et al* (1990)	Structured Clinical Interview for DSM–III–R Dissociative Disorders (SCID–D)	7
Crown & Crisp (1966)	Middlesex Hospital Questionnaire (MHQ)	6.9
Endler *et al* (1962)	Stimulus Response Inventory	6.6
Foa *et al* (1998)	Obsessive–Compulsive Inventory (OCI)	6.0 (42-item inventory that has recently been introduced in shortened form (Foa *et al*, 2002) which may be superseding the original)
Snaith *et al* (1982)	Clinical Anxiety Scale	5.5 (an attempt to compensate for the over-somatic representation of the Hamilton scale)
Gelder & Marks (1966)	Gelder–Marks Phobia Questionnaire	5.1
Bandelow (1995)	Panic and Agoraphobia Scale	5.1
Davidson & Miner (1997)	Brief Social Phobia Scale	5.0
Tyrer *et al* (1984)	Brief Anxiety Scale	4.2 (linked to Comprehensive Psychopathological Rating Scale (CPRS))
Snaith *et al* (1978)	Irritability–Depression–Anxiety Scale (IDA)	3.7 (probably the only measure of irritability available)

Table 14 Scales for the assessment of sleep disorders

Author(s)	Name of scale	Citations per year
Carskadon (1986)	Multiple Sleep Latency Test (MSLT)	30.1
Guilleminault (1982)	Sleep Questionnaire and Assessment of Wakefulness (SQAW)	7.5
Ellis *et al* (1981)	St Mary's Hospital Sleep Questionnaire	3.6
Parrott & Hindmarch (1978)	Sleep Evaluation Questionnaire (SEQ)	3.1
Hoddes *et al* (1972*a,b*)	Stanford Sleepiness Scale (SSS)	3.1

differentiation, as has the focus of psychological treatments on negative symptoms (Sensky *et al*, 2000). Standard scales for the measurement of adverse effects are also included here. The clear preference for the measurement of akathisia is the Barnes scale (1989) and for tardive dyskinesia the Tardive Dyskinesia Rating Scale (TDRS; Simpson, 1988), but there are several competitors for primacy when other abnormal movements are being measured.

Childhood disorders

There are an astonishingly large number of scales in child and adolescent psychiatry; this is as much an expression of wonderment as one of criticism. It is a pity that for so many areas there are no clear preferences or obvious front-runners. For specific areas the scales may select themselves. The Parental Bonding Instrument (PBI; Parker *et al*, 1979) is one such example; it has almost become a *sine qua non* of the assessment of early relational attachment. For other subjects it has become common for scales developed in adult practice to be adapted for children. Well-known examples include the Kiddie–SADS (K–SADS; Puig-Antich & Chambers, 1978) and the Leyton Obsessional Inventory – Child Version (Berg *et al*, 1986; Table 16). There has been considerable recent interest in attention-deficit hyperactivity disorder in children and in the autistic spectrum of disorders, and some recently introduced instruments are likely to be widely used (e.g. Holmes *et al*, 2004; Hansson *et al*, 2005).

When choosing instruments in child psychiatry it is important to ensure that the age range over which the instrument has been validated is the same as the population for which the researcher requires the instrument.

Table 15 Scales for the assessment of schizophrenia and related psychotic disorders (including adverse effects)

Author(s)	Name of scale	Citations per year and comments
Endicott & Spitzer (1978)	Schedule for Affective Disorders and Schizophrenia (SADS)	146.8
Overall & Gorham (1962)	Brief Psychiatric Rating Scale (BPRS)	123.3 (the oldest scale but still has many merits and is likely to be relevant however diagnostic practice changes)
Bernstein & Putnam (1986)	Dissociative Experiences Scale (DES)	44.4
Andreasen (1982a,b)	Scale for the Assessment of Negative Symptoms (SANS)	42.7 (steadily increasing in use as the importance of negative symptoms in treatment outcome grows)
Barnes (1989)	Barnes Akathisia Rating Scale (BARS)	34.1 (the standard scale for recording akathisia)
Andreasen (1984)	Scale for the Assessment of Positive Symptoms (SAPS)	22.5
Andreasen et al (1992)	Comprehensive Assessment of Symptoms and History CASH)	20.7
Simpson (1988)	Tardive Dyskinesia Rating Scale (TDRS)	12.9
Andreasen (1979)	Thought, Language and Communication Rating Scale (TLC)	11.2
Claridge & Broks (1984)	Schizotypy Questionnaire (STQ)	10.6
Birchwood et al (1990)	Social Functioning Schedule (SFS)	5.5 (included here as it was specially prepared for the measurement of social function in schizophrenic patients)
Kendler et al (1983)	Dimensions of Delusional Experience Scale	3.7

Table 16   Scales for the assessment of childhood disorders

Author(s)	Name of scale	Citations per year
Conners (1969)	Conners Rating Scales	33.1
Herjanic & Campbell (1977)	Diagnostic Interview for Children & Adolescents (DICA)	33.1
Parker et al (1979)	Parental Boding Instrument (PBI)	33
Puig-Antich & Chambers (1978)	Kiddie–SADS (K–SADS)	27.2
Kovacs (1985)	Children's Depression Inventory (CDI)	26.3
Reynolds & Richmond (1978)	Revised Children's Manifest Anxiety Scale	26.3
Wechsler (1949)	Wechsler Intelligence Scale for Children	23.3
Achenbach (1978); Achenbach & Edelbrock (1979)	Child Behaviour Check-List (CBCL)	21.7
Puig-Antich et al (1980)	Kiddie–SADS–E (K–SADS–E)	19.9
Ward et al (1993)	Wender Utah Rating Scale (WURS)	18.7
Achenbach & McConaughy (1987a,b)	Empirically-Based Assessment of Child and Adolescent Psychopathology	14
Hodges et al (1982)	Child Assessment Schedule (CAS)	12.4
Harris (1963)	Goodenough–Harris Figure Drawing Test	12.3
Castaneda et al (1956)	Children's Manifest Anxiety Scale (CMAS)	10.1
Birleson (1981)	Depression Self-Rating Scale (DSRS)	9.4
Costello et al (1984)	Diagnostic Interview Schedule for Children (DISC)	7.7
Richman & Graham (1971)	Behavioural Screening Questionnaire (BSQ)	7.2
Berg et al (1986)	Leyton Obsessional Inventory – Child Version	6.2
Poznanski et al (1979)	Children's Depression Rating Scale (CDRS)	6
Carey (1970)	Carey Infant Temperament Scale	5.7
Ambrosini et al (1989)	Kiddie–SADS–III–R (K–SADS–III–R)	5.1
Lefkowitz & Tesing (1980)	Peer Nomination Inventory for Depression	5
Elliott et al (1983)	British Ability Scales – Revised (BAS–R)	4.9
Ullman et al (1984)	ADD–H Comprehensive Teacher Rating Scales (ACTeRS)	4.3
Reynolds et al (1985)	Child Depression Scale (CDS)	4

continued

Table 16 *continued*

Author(s)	Name of scale	Citations per year
Wing & Gould (1978)	Handicap, Behaviour and Skills (HBS)	3.9
Rutter (1967)	Rutter B(2) Scale	3.7
Quay & Peterson (1975)	Behavior Problem Checklist (BPC)	3.3
Zatz & Chassin (1983)	Children's Cognitive Assessment Questionnaire (CCAQ)	2.9
Matson *et al* (1991)	Diagnostic Assessment for the Severely Handicapped (DASH)	2.1

Social and behavioural measurement

The recording of social function is becoming a much more prominent part of measurement generally as it is now realised that functioning is probably more important than symptoms in determining the extent of pathology (Tyrer & Casey, 1993). Whether patients are admitted to hospital, either voluntarily or compulsorily, is determined much more by their general roles in society and their general functioning than by any independent measure of 'illness' *per se*. This is now recognised in multi-axial classification systems, in which social function and disability are given an axis for their domain, and in the growth of scales for recording social function in every medical condition. The scale that is cited more than any other is SF–36, the shortened form of an original medical outcomes scale which is so constructed as to record function in any disorder (Ware & Sherbourne, 1992). It is therefore used in many conditions, which explains its wide usage. It basically comprises one multi-item scale assessing eight health concepts: limitations in physical activities because of health problems; limitations in social activities because of physical or emotional problems; limitations in usual role activities because of physical health problems; bodily pain; general mental health (psychological distress and well-being); limitations in usual activities because of emotional problems; vitality (energy and fatigue); and general health perceptions. Sleep may also be included here. SF–36 is not always ideal for many psychiatric studies but is now such a benchmark measure that it should always be considered if general functioning is being measured.

Table 17 gives a comprehensive list of scales that encompass the range of subjects covered by social function and behaviour. Some of these are highly specific, if not idiosyncratic, but because of the frequent need for a specific instrument all are included.

Table 17 Scales for the assessment of social functioning

Author(s)	Name of scale	Citations per year
Ware & Sherbourne (1992)	Short Form 36 (SF–36) of Medical Outcomes Scale (MOS)	365.5
Holmes & Rahe (1967)	Social Readjustment Rating Scale	107.5
Kanner et al (1981)	Hassles Scale	49.9
Kanner et al (1981)	Uplifts Scale	49.9
Crowne & Marlowe (1960)	Marlowe–Crowne Social Desirability Scale (M–CSDS)	47.8
Sarason et al (1983)	Social Support Questionnaire (SSQ)	35.1
Russell et al (1978)	University of California, Los Angeles Loneliness Scale	30.5
Horowitz et al (1988)	Inventory of Personal Problems	25.8
Weissman & Bothwell (1976)	Social Adjustment Scale Self-Report (SAS–SR)	25.2
Jarman (1983)	Jarman Index	20.1
Paykel et al (1971)	Interview for Recent Life Events	12.5
Vaughan & Leff (1976)	Camberwell Family Interview (CFI)	11.6
Katz & Lyerly (1963)	Katz Adjustment Scale–Relatives Form (KAS–R)	10.6
Honigfeld & Klett (1965)	Nurses' Observation Scale for Inpatient Evaluation (NOSIE)	9.5
Aman et al (1985)	Aberrant Behavior Checklist	8.6
Derogatis (1976)	Psychosocial Adjustment to Illness Scale (PAIS)	8.4
Morosini & Magliano (2000)	Social and Functioning Assessment Scale (SOFAS)	7.9
Henderson et al (1980)	Interview Schedule for Social Interaction (ISSI)	7.9
Wykes & Sturt (1986)	Social Behaviour Schedule (SBS)	7.8
Gurland et al (1972)	Structured and Scaled Interview to Assess Maladjustment (SSIAM)	6.1
Kellner & Sheffield (1973)	Symptom Rating Test (SRT)	6.1
Doll (1965)	Vineland Social Maturity Scale	5.7
Tennant & Andrews (1976)	Life Events Inventory	5.6
Clare & Cains (1978)	Social Maladjustment Schedule (SMS)	4.9
Holmes et al (1982)	Disability Assessment Schedule (DAS)	4.5
Platt et al (1980)	Social Behaviour Assessment Schedule (SBAS)	4.3
Connor et al (2000)	Social Phobia Inventory (SPIN)	4
Margolin et al (1983)	Areas of Change Questionnaire (ACQ)	3.8
McFarlane et al (1981)	Social Relationship Scale (SRS)	3.5

continued

Table 17 *continued*

Author(s)	Name of scale	Citations per year
Jenkins *et al* (1981)	Social Stress and Support Interview (SSSI)	2.9
Tyrer (1990); Tyrer *et al* (2005)	Social Functioning Questionnaire (SFQ)	2.8
Paykel *et al* (1971)	Social Adjustment Scale (SAS)	2.8
Levenstein *et al* (1993)	Perceived Stress Questionnaire (PSQ)	2.8
Hurry & Sturt (1981)	MRC Social Role Performance Schedule (SRP)	2
Olson *et al* (1978)	Family Adaptability and Cohesion Evaluation Scale (FACES)	1.9
Affleck & McGuire (1984)	Morningside Rehabilitation Status Scales (MRSS)	1.9
Baker & Hall (1983)	Rehabilitation Evaluation Hall and Baker (REHAB)	1.8
Linn *et al* (1969)	Social Dysfunction Rating Scale (SDRS)	1.7
Strauss & Harder (1981)	Case Record Rating Scale (CRRS)	1.7
Remington & Tyrer (1979)	Social Functioning Schedule (SFS)	1.7
Schooler *et al* (1979)	Social Adjustment Scale 11 (SAS 11)	1.6
Crandall *et al* (1992)	Undergraduate Stress Questionnaire (USQ)	1.6
Moos (1974)	Ward Atmosphere Scale (WAS)	1.6
Ditommaso & Spinner (1993)	Social and Emotional Loneliness Scale for Adults (SELSA)	1.4
Brugha *et al* (1987)	Interview Measure of Social Relationships (IMSR)	1.4
Cohen & Sokolowsky (1979)	Network Analysis	1.3

Neuropsychological assessment

This is another rapidly expanding area and in most instances there will be a clear indication that will help in the choice of instrument. The measurement of intelligence was one of the first ratings in psychology and it has a worthy tradition in the WAIS, for which special training is required. However, many of the other scales can be used by research trainees but it is wise to seek advice for most of these first as they are not 'off the shelf' instruments (Table 18).

Table 18 Scales for neuropsychological assessment and intellectual disability

Authors	Name of scale	Citations per year and comments
Wechsler (1958)	Wechsler Adult Intelligence Scale (WAIS)	299.9 (the established successor to the early IQ tests; the latest version of this is WAIS–III; Fjordbak & Fjordback, 2005)
Teasdale & Jennett (1974)	Glasgow Coma Scale	98.7
Benton *et al* (1983)	Digit Sequence Learning	50.8
Nelson (1982)	National Adult Reading Test (NART)	46 (a good measure of verbal intelligence that is quick to measure)
Wechsler (1945)	Wechsler Memory Scale (WMS)	38.8
Goodglass & Kaplan (1972)	Boston Diagnostic Aphasia Examination (BDAE)	35.5
Nelson (1976)	Modified Card Sorting Test (MCST)	33.1
Reitan & Davison (1974)	Finger Tapping Test (FTT)	30.8
Benton & Hamsher (1976)	Multilingual Aphasia Examination	18.7
Buschke (1973)	Selective Reminding Test	17.0
Raven (1960)	Raven Progressive Matrices (RPM)	13.5 (an IQ equivalent that can be administered without special training – e.g. by a junior psychiatrist)
Kertesz (1979)	Western Aphasia Battery	12.2
Levin *et al* (1979)	Galveston Orientation and Amnesia Test (GOAT)	9.4
Annett (1967)	Handedness Inventory	8.1 (an established test for lateralisation)
Graham & Kendall (1960)	Graham–Kendall Memory for Designs Test	7.7
Berg (1948)	Wisconsin Card Sorting Test (WCST)	7.4
Banks (1970)	Signal Detection Memory Test (SDMT)	7.2
Warrington & James (1967)	Visual Retention Test (metric figures)	5.1

continued

Table 18 *continued*

Authors	Name of scale	Citations per year and comments
Moss *et al* (1998)	Psychiatric Assessment Schedule for Adults with a Developmental Disability (PAS–ADD) Checklist	5.0 (rapidly becoming a standard screening test for assessment of symptoms in learning disability – is couched in simple language so those without specialised knowledge can readily use the scales)
Thurstone (1944)	Hidden Figures Test	4.2
Armitage (1946)	Trail Making Test (TMT)	3.5
Ferris *et al* (1980)	Facial Recognition and Name –Face Association Test	3.3
Smith (1968)	Symbol Digit Modalities Test (SDMT)	3.3
Dixon (1988)	Metamemory in Adulthood (MIA)	3.2
Lingjaerde *et al* (1987)	UKU (Udvalg for Kliniske Undersolgelser) Side Effect Rating Scale	3.2 (mainly used for detecting adverse effects with antipsychotic drugs)
Holland (1980)	Communication Abilities in Daily Living	3.1

Acknowledgements

We thank Elena Garralda for advice and Sheila McKenzie for secretarial help.

References

Achenbach, T. M. (1978) The child behaviour profile: I. Boys aged 6–11. *Journal of Consulting and Clinical Psychology*, **46**, 478–488.

Achenbach, T. M. & Edelbrock, C. S. (1979) The child behaviour profile: II. Boys aged 12–16 and girls aged 6–11 and 12–16. *Journal of Consulting and Clinical Psychology*, **47**, 223–233.

Achenbach, T. M. & McConaughy, S. H. (1987a) Empirically-based assessment of child and adolescent psychopathology: practical applications. Newbury Park, CA: Sage.

Achenbach, T. M. & McConaughy, S. H. (1987b) Empirically based assessment of behavioural/emotional problems in 2 and 3 year old children. *Journal of Abnormal Child Psychology*, **15**, 629–650.

Adshead, F., Day Cody, D. & Pitt, B. (1992) BASDEC: a novel screening instrument for depression in elderly medical in-patients. *BMJ*, **305**, 397.

Affleck, J. W. & McGuire, R. J. (1984) The measurement of psychiatric rehabilitation status. A review of the needs and a new scale. *British Journal of Psychiatry*, **145**, 517–525.

Aitken, R. C. B. (1969) Measurement of feelings using visual analogue scales. *Proceedings of the Royal Society of Medicine*, **62**, 989.

Alderman, K. J., MacKay, C. J. & Lucas, E. G., *et al* (1983) Factor analysis and reliability studies of the Crown–Crisp experiential index (CCEI). *British Journal of Medical Psychology*, **56**, 329–345.

Alexopoulus, G. S., Adams, R. C., Young, R. C., *et al* (1988) Cornell scale for depression in dementia. *Biological Psychiatry*, **23**, 271–284.

Allen, N. H., Gordon, S., Hope, T., *et al* (1996) Manchester and Oxford Universities Scale for the Psychopathological Assessment of Dementia (MOUSEPAD). *British Journal of Psychiatry*, **169**, 293–307.

Altman, E. G., Hedeker, D. R., Janicak, P. G., *et al* (1994) The Clinician-Administered Rating-Scale for Mania (CARS–M) – development, reliability and validity. *Biological Psychiatry*, **36**, 124–134.

Amador, X. F., Strauss, D. H., Yale, S. A., *et al* (1993) Assessment of insight in psychosis. *American Journal of Psychiatry*, **150**, 873–879.

Aman, M. G., Singh, N. N., Stewart, A. W., *et al* (1985) The aberrant behavior checklist: a behavior rating scale for the assessment of treatment effects. *American Journal of Mental Deficiency*, **89**, 485–491.

Ambrosini, P. J., Metz, C., Prabucki, K., *et al* (1989) Videotape reliability of the third revised edition of the K–SADS. *Journal of the American Academy of Child and Adolescent Psychiatry*, **28**, 723–728.

American Psychiatric Association (1980) *Diagnostic and Statistical Manual of Mental Disorders* (3rd edn) (DSM–III). Washington, DC: APA.

Andreasen, N. C. (1979) Thought, language and communication disorders. I. Clinical assessment, definition of terms and evaluation of their reliability. *Archives of General Psychiatry*, **36**, 1315–1321.

Andreasen, N. C. (1982*a*) Negative symptoms in schizophrenia. *Archives of General Psychiatry*, **39**, 784–788.

Andreasen, N. C. (1982*b*) The scale for the assessment of negative symptoms (SANS). Iowa: University of Iowa.

Andreasen, N. C. (1984) The scale for the assessment of positive symptoms (SAPS). Iowa: University of Iowa.

Andreasen, N. C., Flaum, M. & Arndt, S. (1992) The comprehensive assessment of symptoms and history (CASH). *Archives of General Psychiatry*, **49**, 615–623.

Annett, M. (1967) The binomial distribution of right, mixed, and left handedness. *Quarterly Journal of Experimental Psychology*, **19**, 327–333.

Annis, H. M. (1986) A relapse prevention model for treatment of alcoholics. In *Treating Addictive Behaviors: Processes of Change* (eds W. R. Miller & N. Heather). New York: Plenum Press.

Aquilina, C. & Warner, J. (2004) *A Guide to Psychiatric Examination*. Knutsford, Cheshire: Pastest.

Armitage, S. G. (1946) An analysis of certain psychological tests used for the evaluation of brain injury. *Psychological Monographs*, **60**, 1–48.

Åsberg, M., Perris, C., Schalling, D., *et al* (1978) The comprehensive psychopathological rating scale (CPRS) – development and application of a psychiatric rating scale. *Acta Psychiatrica Scandinavica Supplementum*, **271**, 5–9.

Bandelow, B. (1995) Assessing the efficacy of treatments for panic disorder and agoraphobia 2: the panic and agoraphobia scale. *International Journal of Clinical Psychopharmacology*, **10**, 73–81.

Banks, W. P. (1970) Signal detection theory and memory. *Psychological Bulletin*, **74**, 81–99.

Barnes, T. R. (1989) A rating-scale for drug-induced akathisia. *British Journal of Psychiatry*, **154**, 672–676.

Baron, M., Asnis, L. & Gruen, R. (1981) The schedule for schizotypal personalities (SSP): a diagnostic interview for schizotypal features. *Psychiatry Research*, **4**, 213–228.

Barron, F. (1953) An ego-strength scale which predicts response to psychotherapy. *Journal of Consulting Psychology*, **17**, 327–378.

Barsky, A. J., Wyshak, G. & Klerman, G. L. (1990) The Somatosensory Amplification Scale and its relationship to hypochondriasis. *Journal of Psychiatric Research*, 24, 323–334.

Bech, P. (1993) *Rating Scales for Psychopathology, Health Status and Qualify of Life*. Berlin: Springer.

Beck, A. T., Ward, C. H., Mendelson, M., *et al* (1961) An inventory for measuring depression. *Archives of General Psychiatry*, **4**, 561–571.

Beck, A. T., Weissman, A., Lester, D., *et al* (1974a) The measurement of pessimism: the hopelessness scale. *Journal of Consulting and Clinical Psychology*, **42**, 861–865.

Beck, A. T., Schuyler, D. & Herman, J. (1974b) Development of suicidal intent scales. In *The Prediction of Suicide* (eds A. T. Beck, H. L. P. Resnik & D. J. Lettieri), pp. 45–56. Philadelphia: Charles Press Publishers.

Beck, A. T., Kovacs, M. & Weissman, A. (1979) Assessment of suicidal intention: the scale for suicide ideation. *Journal of Consulting and Clinical Psychology*, **47**, 343–352.

Beck, A. T., Brown, G., Steer, R. A., *et al* (1987) Differentiating anxiety and depression utilizing the cognition checklist. *Journal of Abnormal Psychology*, **96**, 179–183.

Beck, A. T., Epstein, N., Brown, G., *et al* (1988) An inventory for measuring clinical anxiety: psychometric properties. *Journal of Consulting and Clinical Psychology*, **56**, 893–897.

Beecher, H. K. (1959) *The Measurement of Subjective Responses (MSR)*. Oxford: Oxford University Press.

Bell, M. (1981) *Bell Object Relations Self-Report Scale*. West Haven, CT: Psychology Service, VA Medical Center.

Benton, A. L. & Hamsher, K. (1976) *Multilingual Aphasia Examination*. Iowa: University of Iowa.

Benton, A. L., Hamsher K., Varney, N. R., *et al* (1983) *Contributions to Neuropsychological Assessment*. New York: Oxford University Press.

Ben-Tovim, D. I. & Walker, M. K. (1991) The development of the Ben-Tovim Walker body attitudes questionnaire (BAQ), a new measure of women's attitudes towards their own bodies. *Psychological Medicine*, **21**, 775–784.

Berg, C. G., Rapoport, J. L. & Flament, M. (1986) The Leyton obsessional inventory – child version. *Journal of the American Academy of Child Psychiatry*, **25**, 84–91.

Berg, E. A. (1948) A simple objective test for measuring flexibility in thinking. *Journal of General Psychology*, **39**, 15–22.

Bernstein, E. M. & Putnam, F. W. (1986) Development, reliability, and validity of a dissociation scale. *Journal of Nervous and Mental Disease*, **174**, 727–735.

Berrios, G. E., Bulbena, A., Bakshi, N., *et al* (1992) Feelings of guilt in major depression. Conceptual and psychometric aspects. *British Journal of Psychiatry*, **160**, 781–787.

Birchwood, M., Smith, J., Cochrane, R., *et al* (1990) The Social Functioning Scale. The development and validation of a new scale of social adjustment for use in family intervention programmes with schizophrenic patients. *British Journal of Psychiatry*, **157**, 853–859.

Birchwood, M., Smith, J. & Drury, V. (1994) A self-report insight scale for psychosis: reliability, validity and sensitivity to change. *Acta Psychiatrica Scandinavica*, **89**, 62–67.

Birleson, P. (1981) The validity of depressive disorder in childhood and the development of a self-rating scale. *Journal of Child Psychology and Psychiatry*, **22**, 73–88.

Blessed, G., Tomlinson, B. E. & Roth, M. (1968) The association between quantitative measures of dementia and of senile change in the cerebral grey matter of elderly subjects. *British Journal of Psychiatry*, **114**, 797–811.

Brewin, C. R., Wing, J. K., Mangen, S., *et al* (1987) Principles and practice of measuring needs in the long-term mentally ill. *Psychological Medicine*, **17**, 971–981.

Brink, T. L., Yesavage, J. A., Lum, O., *et al* (1982) Screening tests for geriatric depression. *Clinical Gerontologist*, **1**, 37–43.

Broadbent, D. E., Cooper, P. F., Fitzgerald, P., *et al* (1982) The cognitive failures questionnaire (CFQ) and its correlates. *British Journal of Clinical Psychology*, **21**, 1–16.

Brodman, K., Erdnan, A. J., Lorge, I., *et al* (1949) The Cornell medical index. *JAMA*, **140**, 530–540.

Brown, G. & Harris, T. (1978) *The Social Origins of Depression: A Study of Psychiatric Disorders in Women*. London: Tavistock.

Brugha, T. S., Sturt, E., MacCarthy, B., *et al* (1987) The interview measure of social relationships: the description and evaluation of a survey instrument for assessing personal social resources. *Social Psychiatry*, **22**, 123–128.

Bucks, R. S., Ashworth, D. I., Wilcock, G. K. (1996) Assessment of activities of daily living in dementia: development of the Bristol Activities of Daily Living Scale. *Age and Ageing*, **25**, 113–120.

Buglass, D. & Horton, J. (1974) A scale for predicting subsequent suicidal behaviour. *British Journal of Psychiatry*, **124**, 573–578.

Bunney, W. E. & Hamburg, D. A. (1963) Methods for reliable longitudinal observation of behaviour. *Archives of General Psychiatry*, **9**, 280–294.

Burnam, M. A., Karno, M., Hough, R. L., *et al* (1983) The Spanish diagnostic interview schedule. *Archives of General Psychiatry*, **40**, 1189–1196.

Buschke, H. (1973) Selective reminding for analyses of memory and learning. *Journal of Verbal Learning and Verbal Behavior*, **12**, 543–550.

Buss, A. H. & Durkee, A. (1957) An inventory for assessing different kinds of hostility. *Journal of Consulting Psychology*, **21**, 343–348.

Carey, W. B. (1970) A simplified method of measuring infant temperament. *Journal of Pediatrics*, **77**, 188–194.

Carney, M. W., Roth, M. & Garside, R. F. (1965) The diagnosis of depressive syndromes and the prediction of ECT response. *British Journal Psychiatry*, **111**, 659–674.

Carskadon, M. A. (1986) ASDC task force on excessive sleepiness guidelines for multiple sleep latency test (MSLT). *Sleep*, **9**, 519–524.

Castaneda, A., McCandless, B. & Palermo, D. (1956) The children's form of the manifest anxiety scale. *Child Development*, **27**, 317–326.

Chalder, T., Berelowitz, G., Pawlikowska, T., *et al* (1993) Development of a fatigue scale. *Journal of Psychosomatic Research*, **37**, 147–153.

Chambless, D. L., Caputo, G. C., Bright, P., *et al* (1984) Assessment of fear in agoraphobics: the body sensations questionnaire and the agoraphobic cognitions questionnaire. *Journal of Consulting and Clinical Psychology*, **52**, 1090–1097.

Chambless, D. L., Caputo, G. C., Jasin, S. E., *et al* (1985) The mobility inventory for agoraphobia. *Behaviour Research and Therapy*, **23**, 35–44.

Chaney, E., O'Leary, M. & Marlatt, G. A. (1978) Skill training with alcoholics. *Journal of Consulting and Clinical Psychology*, **46**, 1092–1104.

Chick, J. (1980) Alcohol dependence: methodological issues in its measurement; reliability of the criteria. *British Journal of Addiction*, **75**, 175–186.

Clare, A. W. & Cains, V. E. (1978) Design, development and use of a standardised interview to assess social maladjustment and dysfunction in community studies. *Psychological Medicine*, **8**, 589–604.

Claridge, G. & Broks, P. (1984) Schizotypy and hemisphere function – 1: theoretical considerations and the measurement of schizotypy. *Personality and Individual Differences*, **5**, 633–648.

Cohen, C. & Sokolowsky, J. (1979) Clinical use of network analysis for psychiatric and aged populations. *Community Mental Health Journal*, **15**, 203–213.

Cohen-Mansfield, J., Marx, M. & Rosenthal, A. S. (1989) A description of agitation in a nursing home. *Journal of Gerontology*, **44**, M77–M84.

Conners, C. K. (1969) A teacher rating scale for use in drug studies with children. *American Journal of Psychiatry*, **126**, 884–888.

Connor, K. M., Davidson, J. R. T., Churchill, E., *et al* (2000) Psychometric properties of the Social Phobia Inventory (SPIN). New self rating scale. *British Journal of Psychiatry*, 176, 379–386.

Cooper, J. (1970) The Leyton obsessional inventory. *Psychological Medicine*, **1**, 48–64.

Cooper, P. J., Tawor, M. J., Cooper, Z., *et al* (1987) The development and evaluation of the body shape questionnaire. *International Journal of Eating Disorders*, **6**, 485–494.

Cooper, Z. & Fairburn, C. (1987) The eating disorder examination: a semi-structure interview for the assessment of the specific psychopathology of eating disorders. *International Journal of Eating Disorders*, **6**, 1–8.

Conte, H., Plutchik, R., Karasu, T., *et al* (1980) A self-report borderline scale: discriminative validity and preliminary norms. *Journal of Nervous and Mental Disease*, **168**, 428–435.

Copeland, J. R. M., Kelleher, M. J., Kellett, J. M., *et al* (1976) A semi-structured clinical interview for the assessment of diagnosis and mental state in the elderly. I. Development and reliability. *Psychological Medicine*, **6**, 439–449.

Copeland, J. R. M., Dewey, M. E. & Griffiths-Jones, H. M. (1986) A computerized psychiatric diagnostic system and case nomenclature for elderly subjects – GMS and AGECAT. *Psychological Medicine*, **16**, 89–99.

Costello, A. J., Edelbrock, C. S., Dulcan, M. K., *et al* (1984) Development and testing of the NIMH diagnostic interview schedule for children in a clinic population: final report. Rockville, MD: Centre for Epidemiological Studies – National Institute for Mental Health.

Costello, C. G. & Comfrey, A. L. (1967) Scales for measuring depression and anxiety. *Journal of Psychology*, **66**, 303–313.

Cox, J. & Holden, J. (2003) *Perinatal Mental Health: A Guide to the Edinburgh Postnatal Depression Scale*. London: Gaskell.

Cox, J. L., Holden, J. M. & Sagovsky, R. (1987) Detection of postnatal depression. Development of the 10-item Edinburgh Postnatal Depression Scale. *British Journal of Psychiatry*, **150**, 782–786.

Crandall, C. S., Preisler, J. J. & Aussprung, J. (1992) Measuring life event stress in the lives of college students: the undergraduate stress questionnaire (USQ). *Journal of Behavioral Medicine*, **15**, 627–662.

Crown, S. & Crisp, A. H. (1966) A short clinical diagnostic self-rating scale for psychoneurotic patients. The Middlesex Hospital Questionnaire (M.H.Q.). *British Journal of Psychiatry*, **112**, 917–923.

Crowne, D. P. & Marlowe, D. (1960) A new scale of social desirability independent of psychopathology. *Journal of Consulting and Clinical Psychology*, **24**, 349–354.

Cummings, J. L., Mega, M., Gray, K., *et al* (1994) The Neuropsychiatric Inventory: comprehensive assessment of psychopathology in dementia. *Neurology*, **44**, 2308–2314.

Davidson, J. R. T. & Miner, C. M. (1997) Brief social phobia scale: a psychometric evaluation. *Psychological Medicine*, **27**, 161–166.

Davidson, J. R. T., Book, S. W., Colket, J. T., *et al* (1997). Assessment of a new self-rating scale for posttraumatic stress disorder. *Psychological Medicine*, **27**, 153–160.

Derogatis, L. R. (1976) *Scoring and Procedures Manual for PAIS*. Baltimore: Clinical Psychometric Research.

Derogatis, L. R. (1978) Derogatis Sexual Functioning Inventory (DSFI) (revised). Baltimore: Clinical Psychometric Research.

Derogatis, L. R., Lipman, R. S., Covi, L., *et al* (1973) The SCL-90: an outpatient psychiatric rating scale (SCL-90). *Psychopharmacology Bulletin*, **9**, 13–28.

Derogatis, L. R., Lipman, R. S., Rickels, K., *et al* (1974) The Hopkins symptom checklist (HSCL): a self-report symptom inventory. *Behavioral Science*, **19**, 1–15.

Ditommaso, E. & Spinner, B. (1993) The development and initial validation of the social and emotional loneliness scale for adults (SELSA). *Personality and Individual Differences*, **14**, 127–134.

Dixon, R. A., Hultsch, D. F. & Hetzog, C. (1988) The metamemory in adulthood (MIA) questionnaire. *Psychopharmacology Bulletin*, **24**, 671–688.

Dolan, M. & Doyle, M. (2000) Violence risk prediction: Clinical and actuarial measures and the role of the Psychopathy Checklist. *British Journal of Psychiatry*, **177**, 303–311.

Doll, E. A. (1965) *Vineland Social Maturity Scale: Manual of Directions* (revised). Minneapolis: American Guidance Service.

Dupuy, H. J. (1984) The psychological general well-being (PGWB) index. In *Assessment of Quality of Life in Clinical Trials of Cardiovascular Therapies* (eds L. W. Chambers & H. J. Dupuy), pp. 170–183. New York: Le Jacq.

Elliott, C. D., Murray, D. J. & Pearson, L. S. (1983) British ability scales – revised (BAS–R). Windsor: NFER–Nelson.

Ellis, B. W., Johns, M. W., Lancaster, R., *et al* (1981) The St Mary's Hospital sleep questionnaire: a study of reliability. *Sleep*, **4**, 93–97.

Endicott, J. & Spitzer, R. L. (1972) Current and past psychopathology scales (CAPPS): rationale, reliability and validity. *Archives of General Psychiatry*, **27**, 678–687.

Endicott, J. & Spitzer. R. L. (1978) A diagnostic interview: the schedule for affective disorders and schizophrenia (SADS). *Archives of General Psychiatry*, **35**, 837–844.

Endicott, J., Spitzer, R. L., Fleiss, J. L., *et al* (1976) The global assessment scale: a procedure for measuring overall severity of psychiatric disturbance. *Archives of General Psychiatry*, **33**, 766–771.

Endler, N. S., Hunt, J. N. & Rosenstein, A. J. (1962) The stimulus response inventory. *Psychological Monographs*, **76**, 1–33.

Eysenck, H. J. (1971) Personality and sexual adjustment. *British Journal of Psychiatry*, **118**, 593–608.

Ferris, S. H., Crook, T., Clarke, E., *et al* (1980) Facial recognition memory deficits in normal ageing and senile dementia. *Journal of Gerontology*, **35**, 707–714.

Fichter, M. M., Elton, M., Engel, K., *et al* (1989) The structured interview for anorexia and bulimia nervosa (SIAB): development and characteristics of a (semi-) standardised instrument. In *Bulimia Nervosa: Basic Research, Diagnosis and Therapy* (ed. M. M. Fichter), pp. 57–70. Chichester: Wiley.

Fjordbak, T. & Fjordbak, B. S. (2005) WAIS–III norms for working-age adults: A benchmark for conducting vocational, career, and employment-related evaluations. *Psychological Reports*, **96**, 9–16.

Foa, E. B., Kozak, M. J., Salkovskis, P. M., *et al* (1998) The validation of a new obsessive-compulsive disorder scale: The obsessive-compulsive inventory. *Psychological Assessment*, **10**, 206–214.

Foa, E. B., Huppert, J. D., Leiberg, S., *et al* (2002) The Obsessive–Compulsive Inventory: development and validation of a short version. *Psychological Assessment*, **14**, 485–496.

Folstein, M. F., Folstein, S. E. & McHugh, P. R. (1975) "Mini-Mental State": a practical method for grading the cognitive state of patients for the clinician. *Journal of Psychiatric Research*, **12**, 189–198.

Frenken, J. & Vennix, P. (1981) *Sexual Experience Scales Manual*. Lisse: Swets & Zeitlinger.

Fukuda, K., Straus, S. E., Hickie, I., *et al* (1994) The Chronic Fatigue Syndrome – a comprehensive approach to its definition and study. *Annals of Internal Medicine*, **121**, 953–959.

Galissi, J. P., Frierson, H. T. & Sharer, R. (1981) Behavior of high, moderate and low test anxious students during an actual test situation. *Journal of Consulting and Clinical Psychology*, **49**, 51–62.

Garner, D. M. & Garfinkel, P. E. (1979) The eating attitudes test: an index of the symptoms of anorexia nervosa. *Psychological Medicine*, **9**, 273–279.

Garner, D. M., Olmstead, M. P. & Polivy, J. (1983) Development and validation of a multi-dimensional eating disorder inventory (EDI) for anorexia nervosa and bulimia. *International Journal of Eating Disorders*, **2**, 15–34.

Gelder, M. G. & Marks, I. M. (1966) Severe agoraphobia: a controlled trial of behaviour therapy. *British Journal of Psychiatry*, **112**, 309–319.

Gelinas, I. & Gauthier, L. (1999) Development of a functional measure for persons with Alzheimers disease: the Disability Assessment for Dementia. *American Journal of Occupational Therapy*, **53**, 471–481.

Glass, C. R., Merzulli, T. V., Biever, J. L., *et al* (1982) Cognitive assessment of social anxiety: development and validation of a self-statements questionnaire. *Cognitive Therapy and Research*, **6**, 37–55.

Goldberg, D. P. (1972) *The Detection of Psychiatric Illness by Questionnaire (GHQ)*, Maudsley Monograph 21. London: Oxford University Press.

Goldberg, D. P., Cooper, B., Eastwood, M. R., *et al* (1970) A standardised psychiatric interview for use in community surveys. *British Journal of Preventative and Social Medicine*, **24**, 18–23.

Golombok, S. & Rust, J. (1985) The Golombok–Rust inventory of sexual satisfaction (GRISS). *British Journal of Clinical Psychology*, **24**, 63–64.

Goodglass, H. & Kaplan, E. (1972) Assessment of aphasia and related disorders. Philadelphia: Lea & Febiger.

Goodman, W. K., Price, L. H., Rasmussen, S. A., *et al* (1989a) The Yale–Brown obsessive compulsive scale. *Archives of General Psychiatry*, **46**, 1006–1011.

Goodman, W. K., Price, L. H., Rasmussen, S. A., *et al* (1989b) The Yale–Brown obsessive compulsive scale 2. *Archives of General Psychiatry*, **46**, 1012–1016.

Gormally, J., Black, S., Daston, S., *et al* (1982) The assessment of binge eating severity among obese persons. *Addictive Behaviors*, **7**, 47–55.

Gossop, M., Darke, S., Griffiths, P., *et al* (1995) The Severity of Dependence Scale (SDS): psychometric properties of the SDS in English and Australian samples of heroin, cocaine and amphetamine users. *Addiction*, **90**, 607–614.

Gottfries, C. G., Brane, G., Gullberg, B., *et al* (1982a) A new rating scale for dementia syndromes 1. *Archives of Gerontology and Geriatrics*, **1**, 311–330.

Gottfries, C. G., Brane, G. & Steen, G. (1982b) A new rating scale for dementia syndromes. *Gerontology*, **28** (suppl. 2), 20–31.

Graham, F. K. & Kendall, B. S. (1960) Memory-for designs-test: revised general manual. *Perceptual and Motor Skills* (suppl. 2) **11**, 147–148.

Greene, J. G., Smith, R., Gardiner, M., *et al* (1982) Measuring behavioural disturbances of elderly demented patients in the community and its effects on relatives: a factor analytic study. *Age and Ageing*, **11**, 121–126.

Gross, M., Lewis, E. & Nagareijan, M. A. (1973) An improved quantitative system for assessing acute alcohol psychoses and related states (TSA and SSA). In *Alcohol Intoxication and Withdrawal Experimental Studies* (ed. M. M. Gross), pp. 365–376. New York: Plenum Press.

Guilleminault, C. (1982) *Sleeping and Waking Disorders: Indications and Techniques*. California: Addison–Wesley.

Gunderson, J., Kolb, J. & Austin, V. (1981) The diagnostic interview for borderline patients. *American Journal of Psychiatry*, **138**, 896–903.

Gurland, B. J., Yorkston, N. J., Stone, A. R., *et al* (1972) The structured and scaled interview to assess maladjustment (SSIAM). 1. Description, rationale and development. *Archives of General Psychiatry*, **27**, 259–264.

Hachinski, V. C., Iliff, L. D., Zihka, E., *et al* (1975) Cerebral blood flow in dementia. *Archives of Neurology*, **32**, 632–637.

Halikas, J. A., Kuhn, K. L., Crosby, R., *et al* (1991) The measurement of craving in cocaine paitents using the Minnesota cocaine craving scale. *Comprehensive Psychiatry*, **32**, 22–27.

Hall, K. S., Hendrie, H. C., Birttain, H. M., *et al* (1993) The development of a dementia screening interview in two distinct languages. *International Journal of Methods in Psychiatric Research*, **3**, 1–28.

Halmi, K. (1985) Rating scales in the eating disorders. *Psychopharmacology Bulletin*, **21**, 1001–1003.

Halmi, K. A., Falk, J. R. & Schwartz, E. (1981) Binge-eating and vomiting: a survey of a college population. *Psychological Medicine*, **11**, 697–706.

Hamilton, M. (1959) The assessment of anxiety states by rating. *British Journal of Medical Psychology*, **32**, 50–55.

Hamilton, M. (1960) A rating scale for depression. *Journal of Neurology, Neurosurgery and Psychiatry*, **23**, 56–62.

Handelsman, L., Cochrane, K. J., Aronson, M. J., *et al* (1987) Two new rating scales for opiate withdrawal. *American Journal of Drug and Alcohol Abuse*, **13**, 293–308.

Hansson, S. L., Röjvall, A. S., Rastam, M., *et al* (2005) Psychiatric telephone interview with parents for screening of childhood autism – tics, attention-deficit hyperactivity disorder and other comorbidities (A–TAC): Preliminary reliability and validity. *British Journal of Psychiatry*, **187**, 262–267.

Harding, T. W., Arango, M. V. & Baltazar, J. (1980) Mental disorders in primary health care. *Psychological Medicine*, **10**, 231–241.

Hare, R. D. (1980) A research scale for the assessment of psychopathy in criminal populations. *Personality and Individual Differences*, **1**, 111–119.

Hare, R. D. (1991) *The Hare Psychopathy Checklist–Revised*. Toronto, Ontario: Multi-Health Systems.

Harris, D. B. (1963) *Children's Drawings as Measures of Intellectual Maturity*. New York: Harcourt, Brace and World.

Hathaway, S. R. & McKinley, J. C. (1967) *Minnesota Multiphasic Personality Inventory: Manual for Administration and Scoring*. New York: Psychological Corporation.

Hawkins, R. C. & Clement, P. F. (1980) Development and construct validation of a self-report measure of binge eating tendencies. *Addictive Behaviors*, **5**, 219–226.

Helmes, E., Csapo, K. G. & Short, J. A. (1987) Standardization and validation of the multidimensional observation scale for elderly subjects (MOSES). *Journal of Gerontology*, **42**, 395–405.

Helzer, J. E. & Robins, L. N. (1981) Renard Diagnostic Interview. *Archives of General Psychiatry*, **38**, 393–398.

Henderson, M. & Freeman, C. P. (1987) A self-rating scale for bulimia. The "BITE". *British Journal of Psychiatry*, **150**, 18–24.

Henderson, S., Duncan-Jones, P., Byrne, D. G., *et al* (1980) Measuring social relationships: the interview schedule for social interaction. *Psychological Medicine*, **10**, 1–12.

Herjanic, B. & Campbell, W. (1977) Differentiating psychiatrically disturbed children on the basis of a structured interview. *Journal of Abnormal Child Psychology*, **5**, 127–134.

Hersch, E. I. (1979) Development and application of the extended scale for dementia. *Journal of American Geriatrics Society*, **27**, 348–354.

Hoddes, E., Dement, W. C. & Zarcone, V. (1972a) The development and use of the Stanford sleepiness scale (SSS). *Psychophysiology*, **9**, 150.

Hoddes, E., Zarcone, V. & Dement, W. C. (1972b) Cross-validation of the Stanford sleepiness scale (SSS). *Sleep Research*, **1**, 91.

Hodges, K., Kline, J., Stern, L., *et al* (1982) The development of a child assessment interview for research and clinical use. *Journal of Abnormal Child Psychology*, **10**, 173–189.

Hodgson, R. J. & Rachman, S. J. (1977) Obsessional-compulsive complaints. *Behaviour Research and Therapy*, **15**, 389–395.

Hodkinson, H. M. (1972) Evaluation of a mental test score for assessment of mental impairment in the elderly. *Age and Ageing*, **1**, 233–238.

Holland, A. L. (1980) *Communicative Abilities in Daily Living: A Test of Functional Communication for Aphasic Adults*. Baltimore: University Park Press.

Holmes, J., Lawson, D., Langley, K., *et al* (2004) The Child Attention-Deficit Hyperactivity Disorder Teacher Telephone Interview (CHATTI): reliability and validity. *British Journal of Psychiatry*, **184**, 74–78.

Holmes, T. H. & Rahe, R. H. (1967) The social readjustment rating scale. *Journal of Psychosomatic Research*, **11**, 213–218.

Holmes, N., Shah, A. & Wing, L. (1982) The disability assessment schedule: A brief screening device for use with the mentally retarded (DAS). *Psychological Medicine*, **12**, 879–890.

Honigfeld, G. & Klett, C. J. (1965) The nurses' observation scale for inpatient evaluation: a new scale for measuring improvement in chronic schizophrenia. *Journal of Clinical Psychology*, **21**, 65–71.

Hoon, E. F., Hoon, P. W. & Wincze, J. P. (1976) The SAI: an inventory for the measurement of female sexual arousability. *Archives of Sexual Behaviour*, **5**, 291–300.

Hope, T. & Fairburn, C. G. (1992) The present behavioural examination (PBE): the development of an interview to measure current behavioural abnormalities. *Psychological Medicine*, **22**, 223–230.

Horn, J. L., Wanberg, K. & Adams, S. G. (1974) Diagnosis of alcoholism. *Quarterly Journal of Studies on Alcohol*, **35**, 147–175.

Horowitz, L. M., Rosenburg, S. E., Baer, B. A., *et al* (1988) Inventory of personal problems: psychometric properties and clinical applications. *Journal of Consulting and Clinical Psychology*, **56**, 885–892.

Hughes, C. P., Berg, L., Danziger, W. L., *et al* (1982) A new clinical scale for the staging of dementia. *British Journal of Psychiatry*, **140**, 566–572.

Hurry, J. & Sturt, E. (1981) Social performance in a population sample – relation to psychiatric symptoms. In *What is a Case – The Problem of Definition in Psychiatric Community Surveys* (eds J. K. Wing, P. Bebbington & L. N. Robins), pp. 217–222. London: Grant McIntyre.

Hyler, S. E. & Reider, R. O. (1987) *PDQ-R: Personality Diagnostic Questionnaire – Revised.* New York: New York State Psychiatric Institute.

Hyler, S. E., Reider, R. O., Spitzer, R. L., *et al* (1982) *Personality Diagnostic Questionnaire (PDQ).* New York: New York State Psychiatric Institute.

Inouye, S. K., van Dyck, C. H., Spitzer, R. L., *et al* (1990) Clarifying confusion: the confusion assessment method. *Annals of Internal Medicine*, **113**, 941–948.

Jarman, B. (1983) Identification of underprivileged areas. *BMJ*, **286**, 1705–1709.

Jenkins, G., Hale, R., Papassatasiou, M., *et al* (2002) Suicide rate 22 years after parasuicide: cohort study. *British Medical Journal*, **325**, 1155.

Jenkins, R., Maurs, A. H. & Belsey, E. (1981) The background, design and use of a short interview to assess social stress and support in research and clinical settings. *Social Science and Medicine*, **15**, 195–203.

Johnson, C. (1985) Initial consultation for patients with bulimia and anorexia nervosa. In *Handbook of Psychotherapy for Anorexia Nervosa and Bulimia* (eds D. Garner & P. Garfinkel), pp. 19–51. New York: Guilford Press.

Jorm, A. F. & Jacomb, P. A. (1989) The informant questionnaire on cognitive decline in the elderly (IQCODE): socio-demographic correlates, reliability, validity and some norms. *Psychological Medicine*, **19**, 1015–1022.

Jorm, A. F., MacKinnon, A. S., Henderson, A. S. (1995) Psychogeriatric Assessment Scales. A multidimensional alternative to categorical diagnosis of dementia and depression in the elderly. *Psychological Medicine*, **25**, 447–460.

Kandel, D. B. & Davies, M. (1982) Epidemiology of depressive mood in adolescents. *Archives of General Psychiatry*, **39**, 1205–1217.

Kanner, A. D., Coyne, J. C., Schaefer, C., *et al* (1981) Comparison of two modes of stress management: daily hassles and uplifts versus major life events. *Journal of Behavioral Medicine*, **4**, 1–39.

Katz, M. M. & Lyerly, S. B. (1963) Methods for measuring adjustment and social behaviour in the community: 1 Rationale, description, discriminative validity and scale development. *Psychological Reports*, **13** (suppl. 4), 503–555.

Katz, S., Ford, A. B., Moskowitch, R. W., *et al* (1963) Studies of illness in the aged: the index of ADL. *JAMA*, **185**, 914–919.

Katzman, R., Brown, T., Fuld, P., *et al* (1983) Validation of a short orientation-memory-concentration test of cognitive impairment. *American Journal of Psychiatry*, **140**, 734–739.

Keane, T. M., Cadell, J. M. & Taylor, K. L. (1988) Mississippi scale for combat-related posttraumatic stress disorder: three studies in reliability and validity. *Journal of Consulting and Clinical Psychology*, **56**, 85–90.

Kellner, R. (1987) A symptom questionnaire. *Journal of Clinical Psychiatry*, **48**, 268.

Kellner, R. & Sheffield, B. F. (1973) A self-rating scale of distress. *Psychological Medicine*, **3**, 88–100.

Kendell, R. & Jablensky, A. (2003) Distinguishing between the validity and utility of psychiatric diagnoses. *American Journal of Psychiatry*, **160**, 4–12.

Kendler, K. S., Glazer, W. M. & Morgenstern, H. (1983) Dimensions of delusional experience. *American Journal of Psychiatry*, **140**, 466–469.

Kendrick, D. C., Gibson, A. J. & Moyes, I. C. A. (1979) The revised Kendrick battery: clinical studies. *British Journal of Social and Clinical Psychology*, **18**, 329–340.

Kertesz, A. (1979) *Aphasia and Associated Disorders*. New York: Grune & Stratton.

Knopman, D. S., Knapp, M. J., Gracon, S. I., *et al* (1994) The Clinician Interview-Based Impression (CIBI): a clinicians' global change rating scale in Alzheimer's disease. *Neurology*, **44**, 2315–2321.

Kopelman, M., Wilson, B. & Baddeley, A. (1990) *The Autobiographical Memory Interview (AMI)*. Bury St Edmunds: Thames Valley Test Company.

Kovacs, M. (1985) The children's depression inventory. *Psychopharmacology Bulletin*, **21**, 995–998.

Kreitman, N. & Foster, J. (1991) The construction and selection of predictive scales, with special reference to parasuicide. *British Journal of Psychiatry*, **159**, 185–192.

Kuriansky, J. & Gurland, B. J. (1976) The performance test of activities of daily living. *International Journal of Aging and Human Development*, **7**, 343–352.

Larsen, D. L., Attkisson, C. C., Hargreaves, W. A., *et al* (1979) Assessment of client/patient satisfaction: development of a general scale. *Evaluation and Programme Planning*, **2**, 197–207.

Lawton, M. P. (1975) The Philadelphia geriatric center morale scale: a revision. *Journal of Gerontology*, **30**, 85–89.

Lawton, M. P. (1988*a*) Instrumental activities of daily living (IADL) scale: original observer-rated version. *Psychopharmacology Bulletin*, **24**, 785–787.

Lawton, M. P. (1988*b*) Instrumental activities of daily living (IADL) scale: self-rated version. *Psychopharmacology Bulletin*, **24**, 789–791.

Lawton, M. P. & Brody, E. M. (1969) Assessment of older people: self-maintaining and instrumental activities of daily living. *Gerontologist*, **9**, 179–186.

Lawton, M. P., Moss, M., Fulcomer, M., *et al* (1982) A research and service oriented multilevel assessment instrument. *Journal of Gerontology*, **37**, 91–99.

Lefkowitz, M. M. & Tesing, E. P. (1980) Assessment of childhood depression. *Journal of Consulting and Clinical Psychology*, **48**, 43–50.

Levenstein, S., Prantera, C., Varvo, V., *et al* (1993) Development of the perceived stress questionnaire: a new tool for psychosomatic research. *Journal of Psychosomatic Research*, **37**, 19–32.

Levin, H. S., O'Donnell, V. M., Grossman, R. G., *et al* (1979) The Galveston orientation and amnesia test: a practical scale to assess cognition after head injury. *Journal of Nervous and Mental Disease*, **167**, 675–684.

Lewis, G., Pelosi, A. J., Araya, R., *et al* (1992) Measuring psychiatric disorder in the community: a standardized assessment for use by lay interviewers. *Psychological Medicine*, **22**, 465–486.

Lingjaerde, O., Ahlfors, U. G., Bech, P., *et al* (1987) The UKU side effect rating scale: a new comprehensive rating scale for psychotropic drugs and a cross-sectional study of side effects in neuroleptic-treated patients. *Acta Psychiatrica Scandinavica Supplementum*, **334**, 1–100..

Linn, M. W., Sculthorpe, W. B., Evje, M., *et al* (1969) A social dysfunction rating scale. *Journal of Psychiatric Research*, **6**, 299–306.

Litman, G. K., Stapleton, J., Oppenheim, A. N., *et al* (1983) An instrument for measuring coping behaviours in hospitalised alcoholics: implications for relapse prevention treatment. *British Journal of Addiction*, **78**, 269–276.

Litman, G. K., Stapleton, J., Oppenheim, A. N., *et al* (1984) The relationship between coping behaviours, their effectiveness and alcoholism relapse and survival. *British Journal of Addiction*, **79**, 283–291.

Livesley, W. J. (2001) Commentary on reconceptualizing personality disorder categories using trait dimensions. *Journal of Personality*, **69**, 277–286.

Logsdon, R. G. & Gibbons, I. E. (1999) Quality of life in Alzheimer's disease: patient and caregiver reports. *Journal of Mental Health and Ageing*, **5**, 21–32.

Lopiccolo, J. & Steger, J. C. (1974) The sexual interaction inventory; a new instrument for the assessment of sexual dysfunction. *Archives of Sexual Behaviour*, **3**, 585–596.

Loranger, A. W., Susman, V. L., Oldham, J. M., *et al* (1985) *Personality Disorder Examination (PDE): A Structured Interview for DSM–III–R and ICD–9 Personality Disorders – WHO/ADAMHA Pilot Version*. New York: New York Hospital, Cornell Medical Center.

Lorr, M. & Youniss, J. (1983) *The Interpersonal Style Inventory*. Los Angeles: Western Psychological Services.

Lorr, M., McNair, D. M., Michaux, W. W., *et al* (1962) Frequency of treatment and change in psychotherapy. *Journal of Abnormal and Social Psychology*, **64**, 281–292.

Lubin, B. (1965) Adjective checklists for measurement of depression. *Archives of General Psychiatry*, **12**, 57–62.

Luborsky, L. (1962) Clinicians' judgements of mental health: a proposed scale. *Archives of General Psychiatry*, **7**, 407–417.

Mann, A. H., Jenkins, R., Cutting, J. C., *et al* (1981) The development and use of a standardized assessment of abnormal personality. *Psychological Medicine*, **11**, 839–847.

Margolin, G., Talovic, S. & Weinstein, C. D. (1983) Areas of change questionnaire: a practical guide to marital assessment. *Journal of Consulting and Clinical Psychology*, **51**, 920–931.

Markova, I. S. & Berrios, G. E. (1992) The assessment of insight in clinical psychiatry: a new scale. *Acta Psychiatrica Scandinavica*, **86**, 159–164.

Marks, I. M. & Mathews, A. M. (1979) Brief standard self-rating scale for phobic patients. *Behaviour Research and Therapy*, **17**, 263–267.

Marmar, C. R., Horowitz, M. J., Weiss, D. S., *et al* (1986) Development of the therapeutic rating system. In *The Psychotherapeutic Process: A Research Handbook* (eds L. S. Greenberg & W. M. Pinsof), pp. 367–390. New York: Guilford Press.

Marshall, M., Lockwood, A., Bradley, C., *et al* (2000) Unpublished rating scales: A major source of bias in randomised controlled trials of treatments for schizophrenia. *British Journal of Psychiatry*, **176**, 249–252.

Matson, J. L., Gardner, W. I., Coe, D. A., *et al* (1991) A scale for evaluating emotional disorders in severely and profoundly mentally retarded persons. Development of the Diagnostic Assessment for the Severely Handicapped (DASH) scale. *British Journal of Psychiatry*, **159**, 404–409.

Mayfield, D., McLeod, G. & Hall, P. (1974) The CAGE questionnaire: validation of a new alcoholism screening instrument. *American Journal of Psychiatry*, **131**, 1121–1123.

McFarlane, A. H., Neale, K. A., Normal, G. R., *et al* (1981) Methodological issues in developing a scale to measure social support. *Schizophrenia Bulletin*, **7**, 90–100.

McGuffin, P., Farmer, A. E. & Harvey, I. (1991) A polydiagnostic application of operational criteria in studies of psychotic illness: development and reliability of the OPCRIT system. *Archives of General Psychiatry*, **48**, 764–770.

McLennan, A. T., Buborsky, L., O'Brien, C. P., *et al* (1980) An improved evaluation instrument for substance abuse patients: the addiction severity index. *Journal of Nervous and Mental Disease*, **168**, 26–33.

McNair, D. M. & Lorr, M. (1964) An analysis of mood in neurotics. *Journal of Abnormal and Social Psychology*, **69**, 620–627.

Meer, B. & Baker, J. A. (1966) The Stockton geriatric rating scale. *Journal of Gerontology*, **21**, 392–403.

Melzack, R. (1987) The short-form McGill pain questionnaire (SF–MPQ). *Pain*, **30**, 191–197.

Millon, T. (1981) *Disorders of Personality: Axis II.* New York: Wiley.

Mohs, R. C., Rosen, W. G. & Davies, K. L. (1983) The Alzheimer's disease assessment scale: an instrument for assessing treatment efficacy. *Psychopharmacology Bulletin,* **19**, 448–449.

Monahan, J., Steadman, H. J., Silver, E., *et al* (2001) *Rethinking Risk Assessment: The MacArthur Study of Mental Disorder and Violence.* Oxford: Oxford University Press.

Montgomery, S. A. & Åsberg, M. (1979) A new depression scale designed to be sensitive to change. *British Journal of Psychiatry,* **134**, 382–389.

Moos, R. H. (1974) *The Ward Atmosphere Scale Manual.* Palo Alto, CA: Consulting Psychologists Press.

Morey, L. C., Waugh, P. & Blashfield, R. K. (1985) MMPI scales for DSM–III disorders: their derivation and correlates. *Journal of Personality Assessment,* **49**, 245–251.

Morgan, H. G. & Russell, G. F. M. (1975) Value of family background and clinical features as predictors of long-term outcome in anorexia nervosa: four year follow up study of 41 patients. *Psychological Medicine,* **5**, 355–371.

Morosini, P. L. & Magliano, L. (2000) Development of reliability and acceptability of a new version of the DSM–IV Social and Functioning Assessment Scale (SOFAS) to assess routine social function. *Acta Psychiatrica Scandinavica,* **101**, 323–329.

Moss, S., Prosser, H., Costello, H., *et al* (1998). Reliability and validity of the PAS–ADD checklist for detecting psychiatric disorders in adults with intellectual disability. *Journal of Intellectual Disability Research,* **42**, 173–183.

Motto, J. A., Heilbron, D. C. & Juster, J. P. (1985) Development of a clinical instrument to estimate suicide risk. *American Journal of Psychiatry,* **142**, 680–686.

Nelson, H. E. (1976) A modified card sorting test sensitive to frontal lobe defects. *Cortex,* **12**, 313–324.

Nelson, H. E. (1982) *National Adult Reading Test (NART) for the Assessment of Premorbid Intelligence in Patients with Dementia: Test Manual.* Windsor: NFER–Nelson.

Neugarten, B. L., Havighurst, R. J. & Tobin, S. S. (1961) The measurement of life satisfaction. *Journal of Gerontology,* **16**, 134–143.

Nichols, H. & Molinder, I. (1984) *Manual for the Multiphasic Sex Inventory* (MSI). Tacoma, WA: Crime and Victims Psychology Specialists.

Olson, D. H., Bell, R. & Portner, J. (1978) *The Family Adaptability and Cohesion Evaluation Scale (FACES).* St Paul, MN: Family Social Science, University of Minnesota.

Overall, J. E. & Gorham, D. R. (1962) The brief psychiatric rating scale. *Psychological Reports,* **10**, 799–812.

Pallis, D. J., Barrraclough, B. M., Levey, A. B., *et al* (1982) Estimating suicide risk among attempted suicides: 1. The development of new clinical scales. *British Journal of Psychiatry,* **141**, 37–44.

Palmstierna, T. & Wistedt, B. (1987) Staff observation and aggression scale, SOAS: presentation and evaluation. *Acta Psychiatrica Scandinavica,* **76**, 657–673.

Parker, G., Tupling, H. & Brown, L. B. (1979) Parental bonding instrument (PBI). *British Journal of Medical Psychology,* **52**, 1–10.

Parloff, M. B., Kelman, H. C. & Frank, J. D. (1954) Comfort, effectiveness and self-awareness as criteria of improvement in psychotherapy. *American Journal of Psychiatry,* **111**, 343–351.

Parrott, A. C. & Hindmarch, J. (1978) Factor analysis of a sleep evaluation questionnaire (SEQ). *Psychological Medicine,* **8**, 325–329.

Patel, V. & Hope, R. A. (1992) A rating scale for aggressive behaviour in the elderly – the RAGE. *Psychological Medicine,* **22**, 211–221.

Pattie, A. H. & Gilleard, C. J. (1979) *Manual of the Clifton Assessment Procedures for the Elderly* (CAPE). Kent: Hodder & Stoughton.

Paykel, E. S., Prusoff, B. A., Uhlenhuth, E. H., *et al* (1971) Scaling of life events. *Archives of General Psychiatry,* **25**, 340–347.

Pfeiffer, E. (1975) A short portable mental status questionnaire for the assessment of organic brain deficit in elderly patients. *Journal of the American Geriatrics Society,* **23**, 433–441.

Pfohl, B., Stangl, D. & Zimmerman, M. (1983) *Structured Interview for DSM–III Personality*. Iowa: Department of Psychiatry, University of Iowa.

Phelan, M., Slade, M., Thornicroft, G., *et al* (1995) The Camberwell Assessment of Need: the validity and reliability of an instrument to assess the needs of people with severe mental illness. *British Journal of Psychiatry*, **167**, 589–595.

Pilowsky, I. & Spence, N. D. (1975) Patterns of illness behaviour in patients with intractable pain. *Journal of Psychosomatic Research*, **19**, 279–287.

Platt, S., Weymann, A., Hirsch, S., *et al* (1980) The social behaviour assessment schedule (SBAS): rationale, contents, scoring and reliability of a new interview schedule. *Social Psychiatry*, **15**, 43–55.

Plutchik, R., Conte, H., Lieberman, M., *et al* (1970) Reliability and validity of a scale for assessing the functioning of geriatric patients. *Journal of the American Geriatrics Society*, **18**, 491–500.

Plutchik, R., Van-Praag, H. M., Conte, H. R., *et al* (1989) Correlates of suicide and violence risk: 1. The suicide risk measure. *Comprehensive Psychiatry*, **30**, 296–302.

Power, M. J., Champion, L. A. & Aris, S. J. (1988) The development of a measure of social support: the significant others (SOS) scale. *British Journal of Clinical Psychology*, **27**, 349–358.

Poznanski, E. O., Cook, S. C. & Carroll, B. J. (1979) A depression rating scale for children. *Pediatrics*, **64**, 442–450.

Puig-Antich, J. & Chambers, W. (1978) *The Schedule for Affective Disorders and Schizophrenia for School-Age Children*. New York: New York State Psychiatric Institute.

Puig-Antich, J., Orvaschel, H. & Tabrizi, M. A., *et al* (1980) *The Schedule for Affective Disorders and Schizophrenia for School-Age Children–Epidemiologic Version* (3rd edn). New York: New York State Psychiatric Institute & Yale University School of Medicine.

Quay, H. C. & Peterson, D. R. (1975) *Manual for the Behavior Problem Checklist*. Miami, FL: University of Miami.

Qureshi, K. N. & Hodkinson, H. M. (1974) Evaluation of a ten-question mental test in the institutionalised elderly. *Age and Ageing*, **3**, 152–157.

Raistrick, D., Dunbar, G. & Davidson, R. (1983) Development of a questionnaire to measure alcohol dependence. *British Journal of Addiction*, **78**, 89–96.

Raskin, A. & Crook, T. (1988) Relative's assessment of global symptomatology (RAGS). *Psychopharmacology Bulletin*, **24**, 759–763.

Raskin, A., Schulterbrandt, J., Reatig, N., *et al* (1969) Replication of factors of psychopathology in interview, ward behaviour and self report ratings of hospitalised depressives. *Journal of Nervous and Mental Disease*, **148**, 87–98.

Raven, J. C. (1960) *Guide to the Standard Progressive Matrices*. London: H. K. Lewis.

Reisberg, B. (1988) Functional assessment staging. *Psychopharmacology Bulletin*, **24**, 653–659.

Reisberg, B. & Ferris, S. (1988) Brief cognitive rating scale (BCRS). *Psychopharmacology Bulletin*, **24**, 629–636.

Reisberg, B., Ferris, S. H., De Leon, M. J., *et al* (1982) The global deterioration scale for assessment of primary degenerative dementia. *American Journal of Psychiatry*, **139**, 1136–1139.

Reitan, R. M. & Davison, L. A. (1974) *Clinical Neuropsychology: Current Status and Application*. New York: Hemisphere.

Remington, M. & Tyrer, P. (1979) The social functioning schedule – a brief semi-structured interview. *Social Psychiatry*, **14**, 151–157.

Reynolds, C. R. & Richmond, B. O. (1978) What I think and feel: a revised measure of children's manifest anxiety. *Journal of Abnormal Child Psychology*, **6**, 271–280.

Reynolds, W. M., Anderson, G. & Bartell, N. (1985) Measuring depression in childhood. *Journal of Abnormal Child Psychology*, **13**, 513–526.

Richman, N. & Graham, P. (1971) A behavioural screening questionnaire for use with three-year-old children: preliminary findings. *Journal of Child Psychology and Psychiatry*, **12**, 5–33.

Robins, L. N., Helzer, J. E., Croughan, J., *et al* (1981) National Institute of Mental Health diagnostic interview schedule: its history, characteristics and validity. *Archives of General Psychiatry*, **38**, 381–389.

Robins, L. N., Wing, J., Wittchen, H. U., *et al* (1988) An epidemiologic instrument suitable for use in conjunction with different diagnostic systems and in different cultures. *Archives of General Psychiatry*, **45**, 1069–1077.

Robinson, R. G., Parikh, R. M., Lipsey, J. R., *et al* (1993) Pathological laughing and crying following stroke: validation of a measurement scale and a double-blind treatment study. *American Journal of Psychiatry*, **150**, 286–293.

Robson, P. (1989) Development of a new self-report questionnaire to measure self-esteem. *Psychological Medicine*, **19**, 513–518.

Rosenbaum, M. (1980) A schedule of assessing self-control behaviors: preliminary findings. *Behavior Therapy*, **11**, 109–121.

Roth, M., Huppert, F. A., Tym, E., *et al* (1988) *The Cambridge Examination for Mental Disorders of the Elderly (CAMDEX)*. Cambridge: Cambridge University Press.

Ruggeri, M. & Dall'Agnola, R. (1993) The development and use of the Verona Expectations for Care Scale (VECS) and the Verona Service Satisfaction Scale (VSSS) for measuring expectations and satisfaction with community-based psychiatric services in patients, relatives and professionals. *Psychological Medicine*, **23**, 511–523.

Russell, D., Peolau, L. A. & Ferguson, M. L. (1978) Developing a measure of loneliness. *Journal of Personality Assessment*, **42**, 290–294.

Rutter, M. (1967) A children's behaviour questionnaire for completion by teachers: preliminary findings. *Journal of Child Psychology and Psychiatry*, **8**, 1–11.

Salkovskis, P. M., Rimes, K. A., Warwick, H. M. C., *et al* (2002) The Health Anxiety Inventory: development and validation of scales for the measurement of health anxiety and hypochondriasis. *Psychological Medicine*, **32**, 843–853.

Sanavio, E. (1988) Obsessions and compulsions: the Padua inventory. *Behaviour Research and Therapy*, **26**, 169–177.

Sarason, I. G., Levine, H. M., Basham, H. M., *et al* (1983) Assessing social support: the social support questionnaire. *Journal of Personality and Social Psychology*, **44**, 127–139.

Saunders, J. B., Aasland, O. G., Babor, T. F., *et al* (1993) Development of the Alcohol Use Disorders Identification Test (AUDIT): WHO collaborative project on early detection of persons with harmful alcohol consumption II. *Addiction*, **88**, 791–804.

Scheier, M. F. & Carver, C. S. (1985) Optimism, coping and health: assessment and implications of generalised outcome expectancies. *Health Psychology*, **4**, 219–247.

Schooler, N., Hogarty, G. & Weissman, M. M. (1979) Social adjustment scale 11 (SAS 11). In *Resource Material for Community Mental Health Program Evaluators* (ed. W. A. Hargreaves), pp. 290–302. Washington, D.C.: US Department of Health, Education and Welfare.

Schwartz, G. E. (1983) Development and validation of the geriatric evaluation by relative's rating (GERRI). *Psychological Reports*, **53**, 479–488.

Schwartz, R. M. & Gottman, K. M. (1976) Towards a task analysis of assertive behaviour. *Journal of Consulting and Clinical Psychology*, **44**, 910–920.

Sclan, S. G. & Saillon, A. (1996) The behaviour pathology in Alzheimer's disease rating scale. Reliability and analysis of symptom category scores. *International Journal of Geriatric Psychiatry*, **11**, 819–839.

Seligman, M. E. P., Abramson, L. Y., Semmel, A., *et al* (1979) Depressive attributional style. *Journal of Abnormal Psychology*, **88**, 242–247.

Selzer, M. L. (1971) The Michigan alcoholism screening test: the quest for a new diagnostic instrument. *American Journal of Psychiatry*, **127**, 1653–1658.

Sensky, T., Turkington, D., Kingdon, D., *et al* (2000). A randomized controlled trial of cognitive–behavioral therapy for persistent symptoms in schizophrenia resistant to medication. *Archives of General Psychiatry*, **57**, 165–172.

Shader, R. I., Harmatz, J. S. & Salzman, C. (1974) A new scale for clinical assessment in geriatric populations: Sandoz clinical assessment–geriatric (SCAG). *Journal of the American Geriatrics Society*, **22**, 107–113.

Shipley, K., Hilborn, B., Hansell, A., *et al* (2000) Patient satisfaction: a valid measure of quality of care in a psychiatric service. *Acta Psychiatrica Scandinavica*, **101**, 330–333.

Simpson, G. M. (1988) Tardive dyskinesia rating scale (TDRS). *Psychopharmacology Bulletin*, **24**, 803–806.

Skinner, H. A. & Allen, B. A. (1983) Alcohol dependence scale, measurement and validation. *Journal of Abnormal Psychology*, **91**, 199–209.

Skinner, H. A. & Goldberg, A. (1986) Evidence for a drug dependence syndrome among narcotic users. *British Journal of Addiction*, **81**, 479–484.

Slade, P. D. & Russell, G. F. M. (1973) Awareness of body dimensions in anorexia nervosa – cross sectional and longitudinal studies. *Psychological Medicine*, **3**, 188–199.

Slade, P. D. & Dewey, M. E. (1986) Development and preliminary validation of SCANS: a screening instrument for identifying individuals at risk of developing anorexia and bulimia nervosa. *International Journal of Eating Disorders*, **5**, 517–538.

Slade, P. D., Dewey, M. E., Newton, T., *et al* (1990) Development and preliminary validation of the body satisifaction scale (BSS). *Psychology and Health*, **4**, 213–220.

Smith, A. (1968) The symbol digit modalities test: a neuropsychologic test for economic screening of learning and other cerebral disorders. *Learning Disorders*, **3**, 83–91.

Smith, M. C. & Thelen, M. H. (1984) Development and validation of a test for bulimia. *Journal of Consulting and Clinical Psychology*, **52**, 863–872.

Smith, S. G. T., Touquet, R. G. M., Wright, S., *et al* (1996) Detection of alcohol misusing patients in accident and emergency departments: The Paddington alcohol test (PAT). *Journal of Accident & Emergency Medicine*, **13**, 308–312.

Snaith, R. P., Ahmed, S. N., Mehta, S., *et al* (1971) Assessment of the severity of primary depressive illness: the Wakefield self assessment depression inventory. *Psychological Medicine*, **1**, 143–149.

Snaith, R. P., Bridge, G. W. & Hamilton, M. (1976) The Leeds scales for the self-assessment of anxiety and depression. *British Journal of Psychiatry*, **128**, 156–165.

Snaith, R. P., Constantopoulos, A. A., Jardine, M. Y., *et al* (1978) A clinical scale for the self-assessment of irritability. *British Journal of Psychiatry*, **132**, 164–171.

Snaith, R. P., Baugh, S. J., Clayden, A. D., *et al* (1982) The Clinical Anxiety Scale: an instrument derived from the Hamilton Anxiety Scale. *British Journal of Psychiatry*, **141**, 518–523.

Solomon, P. R., Hirschoff, A., Kelly, B., *et al* (1998) A 7 minute neurocognitive screening battery highly sensitive to Alzheimer's disease. *Archives of Neurology*, **55**, 349–355.

Sorgi, P., Ratey, J., Knoedler, D. W., *et al* (1991) Rating aggression in the clinical setting a retrospective adaptation of the Overt Aggression Scale: preliminary results. *Journal of Neuropsychiatry*, **3**, 552–556.

Spanier, G. B. (1987) Measuring dyadic adjustment: new scales for assessing the quality of marriage and similar dyads. *Journal of Marriage and the Family*, **17**, 485–493.

Spiegel, R., Brunner, C., Phil, L., *et al* (1991) A new behavioral assessment scale for geriatric out- and in-patients: the NOSGER (nurses' observation scale for geriatric patients). *Journal of the American Geriatrics Society*, **39**, 339–347.

Spielberger, C. D., Gorsuch, R. L., Luchene, R., *et al* (1983) *Manual for the State–Trait Anxiety Inventory*. Palo Alto, CA: Consulting Psychologists Press.

Spielberger, C. D., Johnson, E. H., Russell, S. F., *et al* (1985) The experience and expression of anger: construction and validation of an anger expression scale. In *Anger and Hostility in Cardiovascular and Behavioural Disorders* (eds M. A. Chesney & R. H. Rosenman), pp. 5–30. Washington: Hemisphere.

Spitzer, R. L, Fleiss, J. L., Endicott, J., *et al* (1967) Mental status schedule: properties of factor-analytically derived scales (MSS). *Archives of General Psychiatry*, **16**, 479–493.

Spitzer, R. L., Endicott, J., Fleiss, J. L., *et al* (1970) The psychiatric status schedules: a technique for evaluating psychopathology and impairment in role functioning. *Archives of General Psychiatry*, **23**, 41–55.

Spitzer, R. L., Williams, J. B. W., Gibbon, M., *et al* (1990a) *Structured Clinical Interview for DSM–III–R – Non-Patient Edition* (SCID–NP, Version 1.0). Washington, DC: American Psychiatric Press.

Spitzer, R. L., Williams, J. B. W., Gibbon, M., *et al* (1990*b*) *Structured Clinical Interview for DSM–III–R – Patient Edition* (SCID–P, Version 1.0). Washington, DC: American Psychiatric Press.

Spitzer, R. L., Williams, J. B. W., Gibbon, M., *et al* (1990*c*) *Structured Clinical Interview for DSM–III–R Personality Disorders* (SCID–II, Version 1.0). Washington, DC: American Psychiatric Press.

Spitzer, R. L., Williams, J. B. W., Gibbon, M., *et al* (1990*d*) *Structured Clinical Interview for DSM–III–R – Patient Edition with Psychotic Screen* (SCID–PW/PSYCHOTIC SCREEN, Version 1.0). Washington, DC: American Psychiatric Press.

Steinberg, M., Rounsaville, B. & Cicchetti, D. V. (1990) Structured clinical interview for DSM–III–R dissociative disorders: preliminary report on a new diagnostic instrument. *American Journal of Psychiatry*, **147**, 76–82.

Steiner, M., Haskett, R. F. & Carroll, B. J. (1980) Premenstrual tension syndrome: the development of research diagnostic criteria and new rating scales. *Acta Psychiatrica Scandinavica*, **62**, 177–190.

Strauss, J. S. & Harder, D. W. (1981) The case record rating scale: a method for rating symptoms and social function data from case records. *Psychiatry Research*, **4**, 333–345.

Stunkard, A. J. & Messick, S. (1985) The three-factor eating questionnaire to measure dietary restraint, disinhibition and hunger. *Journal of Psychosomatic Research*, **29**, 71–83.

Sutherland, G., Edwards, G., Taylor, C., *et al* (1986) The measurement of opiate dependence. *British Journal of Addiction*, **81**, 485–494.

Sunderland, T., Alterman, I. S., Yount, D., *et al* (1988) A new scale for the assessment of depressed mood in demented patients. *American Journal of Psychiatry*, **145**, 955–959.

Tantam, D. (1988) Lifelong eccentricity and social isolation. II: Asperger's syndrome or schizoid personality disorder? *British Journal of Psychiatry*, **153**, 783–791.

Taylor, J. A. (1953) A personality scale of manifest anxiety. *Journal of Abnormal and Social Psychology*, **48**, 285–290.

Teasdale, G. & Jennett, B. (1974) Assessment of coma and impaired consciousness. *Lancet*, ii, 81–84.

Teng, E. L. & Chui, H. C. (1987) The modified mini-mental state (3MS) examination. *Journal of Clinical Psychiatry*, **48**, 314–318.

Tennant, C. & Andrews, G. (1976) A scale to measure the stress of life events. *Australian and New Zealand Journal of Psychiatry*, **10**, 27–32.

Teri, L., Truax, P., Logsdon, R., *et al* (1992) Assessment of behavioural problems in dementia: the revised memory and behaviour checklist. *Psychology and Aging*, **7**, 622–631.

Thurstone, L. L. (1944) *A Factorial Study of Perception*. Chicago: University of Chicago Press.

Trzepacz, P. T., Baker, R. W. & Greenhouse, J. (1988) A symptom rating scale for delirium. *Psychiatry Research*, **23**, 89–97.

Tuckman, J. & Youngman, W. F. (1968) A scale for assessing suicide risk of attempted suicides. *Journal of Clinical Psychology*, **24**, 17–19.

Tyrer, P. (1990) Personality disorder and social functioning. In: *Measuring Human Problems: a Practical Guide* (eds D. F. Peck & C. M. Shapiro), pp. 119–142. Chichester: Wiley.

Tyrer, P. (2001) The case for cothymia: mixed anxiety and depression as a single diagnosis. *British Journal of Psychiatry*, **179**, 191–193.

Tyrer, P. & Alexander, J. (1979) Classification of personality disorder. *British Journal of Psychiatry*, **135**, 163–167.

Tyrer, P. & Casey, P. (eds) (1993) *Social Function in Psychiatry: The Hidden Axis of Classification Exposed*. Petersfield: Wrightson Biomedical.

Tyrer, P., Owen, R. T. & Cicchetti, D. V. (1984) Brief anxiety scale. *Journal of Neurology, Neurosurgery and Psychiatry*, **47**, 970–975.

Tyrer, P., Murphy, S. & Riley, P. (1990) The Benzodiazepine Withdrawal Symptom Questionnaire. *Journal of Affective Disorders*, **19**, 53–61.

Tyrer, P., Jones, V., Thompson, S., *et al* (2003) Service variation in baseline variables and prediction of risk in a randomised controlled trial of psychological treatment in repeated parasuicide: the POPMACT study. *International Journal of Social Psychiatry*, **49**, 58–69.

Tyrer, P., Nur, U., Crawford, M., *et al* (2005) The Social Functioning Questionnaire: a rapid and robust measure of perceived functioning. *International Journal of Social Psychiatry*, 51: 265–275.

Ullman, R. K., Sleator, E. K. & Sprague, R. L. (1984) A new rating scale for diagnosis and monitoring of ADD children (ACTeRS). *Psychopharmacology Bulletin*, **19**, 160–164.

Van Strien, T., Frijters, J. E. R., Bergers, G. P. A., *et al* (1986) Dutch eating behaviour questionnaire for assessment of restrained, emotional and external eating behaviour. *International Journal of Eating Disorders*, **5**, 295–315.

Vaughan, C. F. & Leff, J. P. (1976) The measurement of expressed emotion in families of psychiatric patients. *British Journal of Social and Clinical Psychology*, **15**, 157–165.

Ward, M. F., Wender, P. H. & Reimherr, F. W. (1993) The Wender Utah rating scale: an aid in the retrospective diagnosis of childhood attention deficit hyperactivity disorder. *American Journal of Psychiatry*, **150**, 885–890.

Ware, J. E. & Sherbourne, C. D. (1992) The MOS 36 item short form health survey: conceptual framework and item selection. *Medical Care*, **30**, 473–483.

Warrington, E. K. & James, M. (1967) Disorders of visual perception in patients with localized cerebral lesions. *Neuropsychologica*, **5**, 253–266.

Washton, A. M., Stone, N. S. & Hendrickson, E. C. (1988) Cocaine abuse. In *Assessment of Addictive Behaviours* (eds D. M. Donovan & G. A. Marlatt). London: Hutchinson.

Watson, D. & Friend, R. (1969) Measurement of social-evaluative anxiety. *Journal of Consulting and Clinical Psychology*, **33**, 448–457.

Wechsler, D. (1945) A standardized memory scale for clinical use. *Journal of Psychology*, **19**, 87–95.

Wechsler, D. (1949) *Manual for the Wechsler Intelligence Scale for Children*. New York: Psychological Corporation.

Wechsler, D. (1958) *The Measurement and Appraisal of Adult Intelligence* (4th edn). Baltimore: Williams & Wilkins.

Weissman, M. M. & Bothwell, S. (1976) Assessment of social adjustment by patient self-report. *Archives of General Psychiatry*, **33**, 1111–1115.

Wells, C. E. (1979) Pseudo-dementia. *American Journal of Psychiatry*, **136**, 895–900.

Wilhelm, K. & Parker, G. (1988) The development of a measure of intimate bonds. *Psychological Medicine*, **18**, 225–234.

Wilkinson, I. M. & Graham-White, J. (1980) Psychogeriatric dependency rating scales (PGDRS): a method of assessment for use by nurses. *British Journal of Psychiatry*, **137**, 558–565.

Wing, J. K., Cooper, J. E. & Sartorius, N. (1974) *Measurement and Classification of Psychiatric Symptoms: An Instruction Manual for the PSE and Catego Program*. London: Cambridge University Press.

Wing, J. K., Babor, T., Brugha, T., *et al* (1990) SCAN – Schedules for clinical assessment in neuropsychiatry. *Archives of General Psychiatry*, **47**, 589–593.

Wing, L. & Gould, J. (1978) Systematic recording of behaviours and skills of retarded and psychotic children. *Journal of Autism and Childhood Schizophrenia*, **8**, 79–97.

Wolpe, J. & Lang, P. J. (1964) A fear survey schedule for use in behaviour therapy (FSS). *Behaviour Research and Therapy*, **2**, 27–30.

Wykes, T. & Sturt, E. (1986) The measurement of social behaviour in psychiatric patients: an assessment of the reliability and validity of the SBS schedule. *British Journal of Psychiatry*, **148**, 1–11.

Young, R. C., Biggs, J. T., Ziegler, V. E., *et al* (1978) A rating scale for mania: reliability, validity and sensitivity. *British Journal of Psychiatry*, **133**, 429–435.

Yudofsky, S. C. (1986) The overt aggression scale for the objective rating of verbal and physical aggression. *American Journal of Psychiatry*, **143**, 35–39.

Zahl, D. L. & Hawton, K. (2004) Repetition of deliberate self-harm and subsequent suicide risk: long-term follow-up study of 11 583 patients. *British Journal of Psychiatry*, **185**, 70–75.

Zatz, S. & Chassin, L. (1983) Cognitions of test-anxious children. *Journal of Consulting and Clinical Psychology*, **51**, 526–534.

Zigmond, A. S. & Snaith, R. P. (1983) The hospital anxiety and depression scale. *Acta Psychiatrica Scandinavica*, **67**, 361–370.

Zuckerman, M. (1960) The development of an affect adjective checklist for the management of anxiety. *Journal of Consulting Psychology*, **24**, 457–462.

Zung, W. W. K. (1965) A self-rating depression scale. *Archives of General Psychiatry*, **12**, 63–70.

Zung, W. W. K. (1971) A rating instrument for anxiety disorders. *Psychosomatics*, **12**, 371–379.

Index

Compiled by Caroline Sheard

Printed in the United States
By Bookmasters